The Journey of the Unbreakable Warrior

© 2021, by Mariatu Nyelenkeh
All rights reserved, including the right of reproduction in whole or in part of any form. Printed in the United States of America.
ISBN 978-0-578-96712-7
Library of Congress Catalog Card Number 2021917955
The Journey of the Unbreakable Warrior
Written by: Mariatu Nyelenkeh
Cover Design: Germancreative
Website: www.lupiephoenixx.com

Acknowledgments

Writing a book is harder than I thought it would be. But I wanted the world to hear my story. To be able to see the world I was in. Everything I experienced in my life gave me another outlook. This story is based on true events that took place in my life.

Thank you to my parents, siblings, cousins, and friends for playing a major role in my life when I needed them the most. A special thank you to my children for keeping me sane and placing me in the mindset of reality. Without this group of people, I would not have a story to tell.

I would also like to thank Exposed Books Publishing for allowing me to share my story and showing me the way into the literature world.

Introduction

Can you imagine holding a secret that will get you punished or sent far away from home like Sierra Leone, West Africa? Would you keep that secret if you can? Well, that is what I did at 15 years old, at least until the big secret came out. I was in the 10th grade at District Heights High School. Becoming a teenage mother was the last thing I intended to happen. This is when my journey began and had been going since.

When I was younger, my parents would always threaten to send us away if we were bad in school, disrespectful, or, better yet, get pregnant. When kids are sent away in America, they may go to boarding or military school, even another relative's house. In my household, we were going to another country. I was born and raised in America. If I were going to be shipped away to another country, it would all be a foreign land to me. My parents were from Sierra Leone, West Africa. Their way of growing up was quite different from our upbringing. My mother came to America at age 22 and my father at 26 years old. They came to America to better themselves. My father came first and later sent back home for my mother.

Sierra Leone was known for its precious natural sources like diamonds and rare minerals, but the government was corrupted. The resources that were in Sierra Leone were extremely limited. There was no good healthcare or hospitals. On top of that, it was poverty-stricken and lacked technology. Even with all of that, it is beautiful with deep blue ocean water and white sand beaches. When you say Africa first thing that comes to mind are huts and tigers. This mindset comes from what the media wants you to believe. There are cities and beautiful homes built from concrete.

In 1996 there was an ongoing war in Sierra Leone. This was the same year my parents were taking us to visit. They were cutting children's arms during that war, asking them to choose between short sleeves or long sleeves. I couldn't believe it. This war hit close to home for my family. I lost my grandmother to a stray bullet while she was running for her life. At this time, I was 12 years old, and I received a phone call from my aunt asking to speak with my father. Before I could say anything, my aunt said, "Did you know your grandma died?" When she asked this question, it wasn't in a grieving tone. She was more laughing than anything. My parents were not home at the time. They were at work. I called my mother to inform her of what my aunt said. When I told my mother, she immediately started crying. At 12 years old, I didn't know what to say or do. My mother told me she would call to tell my father. When she called my father to pick her up from work, he was yelling at her. He wanted to know why he was picking her up now when he just dropped her off at work. He thought she might have gotten fired.

I couldn't imagine being in my mother's shoes. How are you supposed to tell your husband his mother died? Do you tell him over the phone or wait until you see him? Before my parents came home, my uncle had arrived there to speak with my father. This was the first time I saw my father bursting out in tears after being told his mother was killed during this war. It was a cry of hurt, frustration, and disappointment. He left her in the care of my great uncle. Sierra Leone was filled with corruption, jealousy, and fighting for land. All of this went on throughout the country between families. There was no way I wanted to risk my freedom by being shipped to a country I am not familiar with. If I did what I was supposed to do, there would be no reason for me to be sent away.

The same year the war took place, we were planning to travel to Sierra Leone. Our trip was canceled. Two years later, we all got on a plane and traveled to my parent's home. There were no direct flights to Sierra Leone. We had three stops on the way there. We stopped in New York, Ghana, Ivory Coast and finally arrived at Lunga Airport. When we got off the plane, there were soldiers, not just adults but kids with guns. Lord, talk about scared. I guess that's what's expected right after a war. We took a ferry from Lunga into the capital Freetown. While I was on the ferry boat, I thought I was going to die. It was rocking back and forth very hard. My sister was throwing up from being seasick. And I was a nervous wreck. I felt sorry for my mother because she was traveling with all three of us, and each of us had two boxes per person plus a carry-on. The one thing about Africans is they never travel light when they are going to their home country. In total, there were eight boxes fully packed with four carry-ons. When we finally arrived at the airport, my uncle had a driver pick us up, and that ride was bumpy as hell. The city was crowded due to everyone coming into Freetown from the war. But it was nothing like what the media showed. I always remembered seeing the commercials of starving children and run-down homes. I was able to see for myself what Africa was like. Sierra Leone, in particular, was full of people just like in America. Everyone wasn't starving, and not all homes were run-down. It was no different than the country I was born in. One of the big differences was Sierra Leone's buildings and houses were built out of concrete.

The first night I was there, I could not sleep. We had to sleep with the mosquito net around the bed. When I finally dosed off, I felt something crawling up my leg and went off! I started screaming for dear life. I don't know what was going through my mind, but I was scared. They just had a war! Come to find out; it was my little cousin who slept badly. I thought it was the Craw Craw Devil my cousin told me about or someone trying to get me. But that was all just my imagination. After a few days of being there, I did not want to go anywhere because

I was afraid. There was nothing to be afraid of. This was just all new to me.

One day my grandmother, who I met for the first time, asked what I wanted to eat, and I told her chicken and salad. To me, chicken and salad is a normal meal. In Sierra Leone, it goes beyond normal. While I was outside playing card games with my cousins in the yard, I saw them boiling water, but my cousin was chasing the chicken around. I figured he was playing with him. I didn't put two and two together. When he finally caught it, they cut the chicken neck right in front of me. I screamed out, "Murderer." My aunt said, "I thought you wanted us to fix you chicken." I responded with, "Yes, I did, but that was before you killed it in front of me." For the remaining two weeks of the trip, I did not want to eat my cultural food. I ate things like bread, chips, dry cereal, and things that I didn't see being killed. Overall, the experience of being able to go to my roots was filled with mixed emotions. I felt fear, but on the other hand, it was astounding, memorable, and educational. I enjoyed myself, but it's not where I can live. When we returned home to America, I knew I would try my best not to make those threats true. But little did I know I had an untold journey ahead of me.

Atu

When I first attended Grayland Middle School in 1997, I did not know anyone because that was not the original school I was supposed to attend. This is where I gained my wings of being a rebel. This was a different neighborhood and set of kids in one school. Time went on, and I started to make friends through classes, lunch, and on the school bus. This is where I met my best friend Zion, Calvin, my play brothers, and Tiana, my so-called friend. I found out later Tiana wasn't my friend.

It was the three Amigos. That's how I saw it, myself, Zion, and Calvin. Those were my boys. I always had their back, just like they had mine. I was the only female in my group besides my god sister Mimi who was five years younger than me. I was not just looking out for them but all the guys we hung out with. When they had female issues, I was the first person they called. It was either hook me up or beat their ass. If they wanted me to do something, I did it. No questions asked. These were my brothers, so there was no need to. If I felt like it later, questions were asked. Out of everyone, I never questioned Zion and Calvin's loyalty because if there was anything I needed or wanted, I had it. Calvin was the shit talker out of us. He always had something to say, but he had a big heart. And not to mention the most sensitive. At the same time, Zion was the go with the flow, mellow, and advisor type. I just knew it would always be us, no matter what.

All of us rode the same bus to school because we lived in the same neighborhood. On the first day of school, all the students were directed to the gym to get their classes. While sitting in the gym waiting for my name to be called, this light-skinned, handsome boy walks up to me and asks me my name. The first thing that went through my mind was, "Mariatu, you don't know anything about boys." I started to have a tingling feeling which was unusual. Here I was entering middle school, and on the first day, this fine light skin, short, and goofy boy is asking for my name. He was standing in front of me, trying to carry on a conversation by joking with me. I was not ready for whatever was to come my way when it came to having feelings for boys. I didn't take this boy seriously. I looked at it as a boy and girl becoming friends. The one thing about him was he always made me laugh. My new friend was goofy. He was known for his dancing and being a clown. I didn't suspect it at the time, but he became my man in the future.

My new friend, Joshua, came with trouble. These girls were boy crazy about him, but this one girl, Star, was my problem. One day we went on a field trip to Pennsylvania. We were seated on the bus by our last name, so Joshua and I were not on the same bus. In the middle of the drive, we made a rest stop to get food and use the restroom. When I stepped off the bus, I was happy to see Joshua until I saw him approach me with Star on his arm. He stood in front of everyone and said, "I don't want to go with you anymore." Without an explanation, Joshua walked away. That was my first heartbreak. All of this was new to me. I still didn't know anything about boys and definitely didn't know anything about having a broken heart. I could not talk to my mother about this. She would kill me. And my father was out of the question, so I kept it to myself and went on with my life.

During middle school, I started looking out for Tiana. We were close, but I found out later I couldn't trust her. I started to question her motives because she was always trying to fit in. Tiana was the reason I got into some of the fights I was involved in. Tiana tried to be about that fight life, but she wasn't built for it. I was such a loyal friend that I would fight for her and not know the story behind the fights half of the time. I was still the person that would react first and ask questions later.

I remember when she was having issues with a group of girls who called themselves PGG "Pretty Girl Gang." Star was part of this group along with two other girls. Tiana had an issue with one of the girls named April. April was dating Tiana's ex-boyfriend. I wasn't sure what happened or why it even got this far, but I protected my friend. I ended up involved because April was a big girl, and I couldn't let anyone bully my friend. They wanted to fight Tiana, so we met up at school early in the morning during breakfast. I wanted to see what the issue was. It all came down to a bunch of non-sense over this boy. One of the girls involved was Star. I already despised Star, so there was nothing much to say.

Tiana's ex-boyfriend decided to play on my house phone. When my mother answered the phone, they called her out of her name. They referred to her as an "African Bitch." They didn't call once or twice. But they continued to play on my phone and kept calling my parents out of their name. This has become personal and was no longer about Tiana. This had become a whole different game. I was going to handle this my way.

At this point, I felt like I had no control over my emotions, thoughts, or even body. I was not thinking at all. I was just ready to hurt her and anyone else involved with disrespecting my parents. I wanted her to know how it felt when you decided to disrespect the people I love. When I got to school, I only told Joshua that I brought a knife to school. I didn't bring a pocket knife, butter knife, or small knife but a big butcher knife. I thought I could trust him. Before I knew it, the 8th-grade class was aware of what I had. The news got back to the principal, and my locker was searched. I thought I would go to juvie, but the knife was no longer in my locker when they checked it. Joshua had gone into my locker, removed the knife, and put it in his. I thought he had disappointed me, but he did not. He may have run his mouth, but he got me out of this one. I was only out of trouble with the knife, but I still felt like hurting this girl. This gave me more time to think.

The end of the day arrived, and Joshua placed the knife back in my book bag. On our way home from school, I went after April's boyfriend because we lived in the same neighborhood. He was a part of the disrespect, and I wouldn't let him get away with it. I took off once the bus stopped and chased him down to his house to his front door. I never caught him, but I banged on his door and disrespected his mother by calling her a "bitch." Did it make me feel better? No, I still felt the same, but he knew not to mess with me.

Later, that evening I received a knock on my door by the principal, April, and her mother. They wanted to speak with my parents due to this situation. I'm thinking, "Oh, now this chic is not big and bad anymore." She had the nerve to bring her mother and the principal to my house. This girl made herself look so innocent that she deserved a Grammy. The principal told us I had to apologize and agree that this will be over between us. April's mother thought she could just easily get an apology out of me, but it was not that easy. But of course, my mother just sat there and agreed to the terms. I did apologize to avoid whatever plans were coming along with me disagreeing. But I will never forget! This is when I was never the same and had to keep up with how I was presenting myself.

These thoughts of reacting when someone did something to me did not occur unless you hurt me or someone like my parents or siblings. It was my mode of protection. When I bottled up all my feelings, the rebel gained her wings and was born. I had to start going to a counselor to talk about my problems and what was bothering me. It was a waste of time. I didn't feel any connection, but I went to keep everyone quiet.

Joshua and I were off and on through middle school. We continued to see each other in the summer because his sibling's father lived across the street from me. It was the summer of 2001, and I was getting ready for high school. On this particular day, everyone was outside. In my neighborhood, we had a tradition and a big day called "Cheverly Day." This is when there is a big basketball game tournament, cookout food, games, and everyone was out.

There was this girl that lived in the building next to me. Her name was Shanae, and she was built like someone from the WWE. This girl had muscles, and when we were at the pool, she did sit-ups by hanging her legs from the poolside lifting her weight up. Supposedly, she was out for me this day. I didn't know why but I heard it could have been because of this boy named Shawn that we knew or people saying she couldn't beat me. After Cheverly Day, everyone was hanging outside; even Joshua was around my way. Shanae knocked on my door, asking for me to come outside. My cousin Eisha was over this weekend. She answered the door when Shanae came to ask for me. Before going outside, she begged me not to go and said this would not be a good decision. But I still chose to go.

When we got outside, everyone was out there waiting as if they knew what was getting ready to happen. Shanae told me she wanted to fight me. I never turned down a challenge, and I wasn't going to start that day. We squared up in the grass at the building next to mine. I swung on her first. I was winning and giving it my all. So, I thought, I wasn't worried about losing this fight. I refused to lose in front of my neighborhood and boyfriend. They were counting on me.

I fell to the ground, and she got on top of me. She started pounding me in my stomach with a rock. I managed to get back up. I was ready to go again. While we were fighting, I didn't feel any pain. I believe it was due to all the adrenaline I

9

was feeling. I soon realized once I stood up that I was weak and could not go for round two. This was something I was going to have to face and live with. This was the first loss and the only loss that I had. I found out later Calvin was the mastermind behind this fight. Shanae and Calvin had a misunderstanding, and she threatened to get her boyfriend. I mean, who else was Calvin going to get to do the dirty work other than me? That is just what we did for each other. Honestly, I think she knew what she was doing, which was her way of calling me out.

New World

My Unpredictable Journey started at District Heights High in 2001 as a 9th grader. When I entered high school, I only knew people from middle school and my neighborhood. On the first day, I was tough on the outside and scared as hell on the inside. But I couldn't show anyone that I was afraid. It didn't take long to make new friends at all. As I made new friends, I had to keep up with my popularity and what I was known for.

There was a group of girls that I met through some of my classes. We were majorettes together. I never saw myself as a majorette. I always considered myself as being stiff, but shit, I had rhythm. We all became close. But that didn't last long. We were a circle within a circle. We ended up having misunderstandings. It was the typical; he said she said drama and boy issues. I never once regretted making friends with them, and honestly, I wish it would have worked out. I felt like I was misunderstood, but I was just being myself, and communication didn't exist in my vocabulary.

During my 9th grade year, I had a boyfriend named CJ. He was popular and was from around Chapel Oaks. His neighborhood was across the street from our school. CJ was another Joshua. The difference between the two was CJ was the prince of females chasing after him. He was pigeon toe, with brown chocolate mocha skin, pretty hair, and big lips. CJ had to keep up with me eventually. I was treating him the same way he was treating other females. My downfall was I couldn't control my emotions. CJ was the reason I was no longer friends with the girls from the majorettes. He was the reason for our friendship ending. There was so much commotion within the group because of him. I didn't know, but one of the girls in the group dated him before we attended District Heights, but they broke up before I met them.

When we started dating, I had no idea he had dated one of my new friends. Once I was aware it was too late, we were already together. I thought she was cool with it, but those were just words out of her mouth. She was in love with him, and I can see he was too. CJ decided to do the back and forth with us. Not only that, but he was too friendly with the rest of the girls in the group. We all started together, but we didn't end together.

I was known to portray a certain image. The same way I was in my neighborhood, I had to be that way in school. One day there was this big fight between the guys in two different neighborhoods. It was Cheverly Terrace and Cherryhill against each other. One day, these older guys from around my way came to my school and some from the other neighborhood. A normal person would have gotten out of the way and stayed out of the hallways. Instead, I wanted to know what was going on, so I stuck around. To be honest, I wanted to make sure I was not needed just in case any females were involved. It was none of my business, but that was the image I had to keep up with. On this day is when my world changed. I met the donor of my son. We were standing face to face.

I had heard of him before, but we never had an encounter until this day. We met in the hallway in the middle of some commotion. When he spoke to me, I started blushing. If you could see the color of my cheeks, they were bloodshot red. He asked for my number, but I told him to give me his. I knew that my father would hang up on him if he were to call my house.

My parents worked on Friday nights, and I was responsible for my brother and sister. When they went to work on Fridays, the party was just beginning. It wasn't a party, but I always had a few people over at my house. One Friday, it was just one of my girlfriends that came over. While we were in the house, there was a knock at the door. It was this guy named

Bryson, and guess who the hell else was with him? It was the future sperm donor. I stood in the doorway and almost pissed my pants. I let them both in. I didn't know what else to do. This was the first time I hung out with an older guy. He was four years older than me. Being in direct contact with someone that had more experience with me was scary.

We hung out and talked for a bit while we were sitting on my balcony. We were getting to know each other. The donor wanted some privacy, so he asked if we could go to the bathroom. My stupid ass fell for the bullshit. We ended up in my bathroom, and I was bent over the bathtub. It felt good at the time, but I was asking myself, "What the fuck are you doing?" While I was getting penetrated, I started to cry. When it was over, I acted like everything was okay. I was good at hiding my feelings. Not only did I have sex with this man that I just met, but he didn't have on a condom. This was the day when my beautiful baby boy was conceived.

After this encounter, there was another side that came out of me. I started doing stuff I wouldn't normally do. I was skipping school and having sex regularly. In my eyes, having sex, making love, and fucking are all different. When you have sex with someone, it should be gentle or enjoyable; both parties involved should feel the outcome. Making love is passionate, hot, steamy, and there's a connection. It's done with feelings and involves someone you love or are in love with. Fucking sums it up to a bunch of hard-ass penetration. It can be with a friend with benefits or whomever without feelings. So which category do you think I was in? I was in the fucking category. In my eyes, I thought that he cared about me, but it was only one thing that I was getting out of this image of a fantasy, a hard dick. We had sex at my house twice. The other times were at his grandmother's house, my best friend's house, in the park, the woods, behind the apartment building, and the famous laundry room. He didn't give two fucks about me, but he played a good game. The donor was so manipulative.

We started to hang tough daily, but mother nature hadn't touched down. It has been a month, and still no sign of her. I was so damn scared that I would still wear a pad. When I realized my period was not showing up, I started putting ketchup on the pads after taking it off and wrapping it up in tissue. I know it may sound crazy, but I had to do what was needed to be done. I refused to be shipped to a country I did not grow up in and possibly getting killed on the way there. Hell no! The only reason why I got away with the moves I was making was because both of my parents worked hard. My mother was in nursing school and could only work on the weekend, and my father worked a lot. They both came home at the same time at night.

That one month has now become a few months that mother nature had not shown up. I was officially pregnant! I may have been 15 years old, but I also knew what it meant when you did not see your period. I didn't take a test because I already knew the deal. I spotted for a few times, but it was very light. I knew my body, and I can tell it was going through some changes that I had never experienced. I started to freak out. I didn't know who I could trust with my newfound secret. I didn't know what to do. What I did know was, I couldn't bring a baby into this world. Not only was I broke, but I have African parents. I started taking pills such as Excedrin, Tylenol, and any other type of pain medication. The plan was to end this pregnancy on its own. At least that was my intention.

As I was trying to end my pregnancy, I was still having sex with the sperm donor. We would hang out at my Zion's uncle's house or the basketball court. Even though I saw him almost every day, I never told him I was pregnant. I didn't know how to bring it up. There were some things I wasn't aware of when it came down to the donor. He was in a situation that was unbeknownst to me. I found out he was engaged and had a baby on the way.

I was still attending school like things were normal. I didn't gain any weight in the stomach, but my feet and face were swollen. I was fat as hell everywhere but my stomach. The kids at my school would ask me if I was pregnant. I would lie and tell them I was on birth control. I still couldn't tell anyone my secret. I was in the 10th grade now, and the one friend I thought I could confide in wasn't there anymore. Our friendship ended when she went to another school. She was one of the girls that I was in the majorettes with. Before everything went down, she was always over at my house. I know she would have kept my secret. I learned early that you couldn't expect "friends" to treat you the same way you would treat them.

I finally decided to let the cat out of the bag about me being pregnant. I told the sperm donor. I was over how he was carrying the shit out of me. There were always other females pulling up on him when I was around. This fool would sleep with anything walking. I was sharing him with the world, and I continued to have sex with him. The day I decided to tell him, it was raining like cats and dogs. I walked to his grandmother's house to give him the big news. After walking in the rain and being soaked, I arrived at his grandmother's house. Before I could tell him, he asked me if I was pregnant. I told him I was. I thought I would finally feel a sense of relief. This moment was the beginning of a nightmare. He let me know I couldn't have the baby because his fiancé was also pregnant. The expression on my face was, "what bitch." I wanted to murder him. My heart was now ice-cold, and there was all kind of thoughts going through my head. I couldn't blame anyone but myself. I knew he didn't care anything about me, but I kept dealing with him. The same way I carried myself in the streets is how I should have carried myself with him. I should have set standards.

I didn't have any money to pay for an abortion. Did he expect me to pay for it? Or was he willing to pay for it? Little did he or anyone else know, I was depressed and possibly suicidal. I was capable of anything and was not afraid of what may come. I was already taking painkillers like Skittles. I left his grandmother's house with no umbrella, not even a hat covering my head. I was walking in the rain. I was distraught with fucked up thoughts in my mind. I was figuring out a way to retaliate. I couldn't go home like this, so I went to Zion's uncle's house.

We called his uncle Pop. When I arrived at Pop's house, I confessed to Zion that I was pregnant. Zion knew the donor was engaged and had a baby on the way. I felt betrayed by my best friend. Zion knew I was having sex with him and didn't tell me about his situation. That was fucked up in my mind. I wasn't sure if Calvin was aware of it at the time. The way Calvin's mouth was set up, he would have told me without holding anything back. Calvin was hard on me, so I believe he would have let me know. I couldn't trust anyone at this point, and I hated the sperm donor guts. I didn't understand why he used me or treated me this way. Maybe it was because I was young, and he knew I didn't have much experience. After leaving Zion's house, my mind was racing. I was in an "I don't give a fuck mood." I was about to play the game the same as him. I knew I had to get out of this situation soon.

This was a big challenge for me with keeping a secret and maintaining my profile. This was the hardest thing I had to do in my life. I continued playing basketball, double dutch, dancing, and still faking it like my period was coming. I was still thought of as the girl with the defendant belt, meaning I was known not to be messed with. I couldn't beat everybody, but I was nobody's bitch for sure. I was never scared of anything.

If you want to be technical, I started fighting in 5th grade on the block top. On the first day of school, we were standing in line by the letter of our last name. One of the girls thought she could cut in front of me because she was taller than me. Height didn't mean anything to me. Just because I was little didn't mean you could mess with me. We began to push each other; then, we started to fight. I was fighting in a wrap skirt, black shirt, and Chinese sleepers. I beat her big ass on the black top in a skirt. The teacher had to grab me off her. She knew not to cut in front of me next time. During the same school year, I felt like my teacher tried to embarrass me in front of the class. I got mad and threw the chair at him. I was filled with anger, but overall, I was a good child.

It seemed like I always involved myself in unnecessary drama. Most of the time, it was because I was trying to save Tiana. On one occasion, there was this girl named Destiny. For some reason, she started coming around my neighborhood thinking she could intimidate me. Destiny probably intimidated some because she was built like Debo from Friday. But she placed no fear in my heart. I couldn't be shaken even though I was undercover pregnant. This all started because Tiana and her cousin Shaniqua were being messy. Tiana started to change as we got older and would act like she did not know me when we would be in school. This would only happen when her cousin Shaniqua was around. I don't know why I continued to be friends with her because I still questioned her loyalty. Shaniqua was telling Destiny things. It was like Tiana was her puppet, and Shaniqua was pulling her strings. I ended up getting pulled under the bus.

One day during lunch, something was about to go down in school, and I had no clue what would occur. I was using the pay phone in the cafeteria when Destiny approached me as if we were in county jail and she wanted to use the phone. I hung up from my call, and I found myself surrounded by about six to eight chicks. The only thing I could think of was how was I going to whip these bitch's ass, what to grab, and who the hell was going to get it first? I was code red with a lot on my mind. I wasn't to be fucked with at that moment. They all found out that day.

Destiny opens her mouth and says, "I want to fight you, but I'm not going to fight you. I'm going to get Brittany to do it." Brittany jumps in with, "I'm not going to fight her." Since no one wanted to step to me, I was going to choose for them. Shaniqua was the instigator. I was standing there with Destiny and Brittany in between me. I was going after Shaniqua. My fist was in the process of making its way to Shaniqua's face, and unfortunately, others met my fist in route. I beat that bitch ass in front of the whole cafeteria that day. Students were standing on the lunch tables and gathering around to see what was going on.

Tiana, who I was defending, grabbed me along with my favorite Vice-Principal. Even with them grabbing me, Shaniqua was already exposed. Her breast was out, and she was beyond fucked up. I took all of my anger out on her. The last thing anyone wanted to do was mess with me on that level. I didn't care that I was pregnant. I did get suspended from school for a week which I got away with because my parents never found out. Trust me; I was good at what I did. I called my godmother, who came to save me, and she pulled me out of the dirt. I went to her house the week I was suspended as if I was going to school.

There's a funny story behind my godmother and me. She had two children who were Kendell and Mimi. Kendell and I were closer in age. We attended Grayland Middle School and District Heights together. Kendell was also a ladies' man. All the girls wanted him, and guess what? Girls would befriend me to

18

get to him. Mimi was a little me. She was the other girl that was in our neighborhood known to fight. We were the go-to when the boys would have girl troubles in our neighborhood. There were situations when we fought mothers and aunts together. There was an incident when we took a girl's snacks behind my building. That was when I realized that we were bullies.

I would always do both my godmother's and Mimi's hair. See, back in the 2000s, when we did hair, it wasn't feed-ins, lace fronts, or frontals. We started from the top and made it look good. I was so good at the time that I did Mimi's hair for her 5th-grade graduation. My parents never gave me godparents. That title was given because of the relationship that Kendell, Mimi, and I had. I could talk to my godmother about anything without judgment. She trusted me when it came to Mimi especially, but she knew that we would protect one another. Unfortunately, when I was in the 10th grade, my godmother had a stroke and eventually passed away right after. I never went to her funeral, not even her grave site. I was afraid to face the fact that she was no longer here, and I had no clue how to show it. Death was something I did not know how to deal with.

Time had passed, and everything was flying by. I didn't know how far along I was. I wasn't showing, no doctor appointments, and I wasn't taking any vitamins. One day I was sitting home with my mother, and she asked me, "Are you having sex?" Damn, I felt like I was about to shit myself. I was scared out of my mind.

I replied, "No."

"Are you sure you aren't having sex?" she continued to question me.

"Yes, I'm sure."

My mother and I only had one discussion regarding sex, and that was when I first had my period in 5th grade. It was brief, nothing serious. She trusted me and didn't think I would be having sex at 15 years old. My mother's expectations were for me to go to church, school and respect my parents. After I answered her final question, she said, "I'm going to make an appointment with your doctor to be checked." My mother said all of this while checking my ankles. The only words that came out of my mouth were, "Okay." Inside I was screaming for help and telling myself I would get shipped off, live on the streets, or better yet, die at the hands of my father. Two days later, my mother took me to the doctor.

All kinds of thoughts were going through my head. I was feeling scared. I thought about running. I wanted someone to kill me. The nurse called my name to the back to be seen. Before anyone could say anything, my mother opened her mouth and said, "Yes, I want my daughter to take a pregnancy test." Without question, the nurse handed me a cup to pee in. The doctor came in to examine me and to check my blood pressure.

I didn't know what Dr. Brown was going to say. He said, "Wow, your blood pressure is extremely high. You have a lot of fluid in your ankles." That was the least of my worries. My concern was the test results. After what seemed like forever, the results came back, and they were negative. I was wondering if Dr. Brown really did her job. Did she do a full exam? Or maybe there was no baby inside of me. Dr. Brown prescribed me this medicine called Naproxen. This was a life saver. My test came back negative, but that didn't stop my mother from watching my every move.

It was February 18, 2002, Presidents Day, and school was closed. My mother was off this day also. I woke up that morning, and everything was black. I mean pitch black dark.

There was no color at all. I figured I was still sleepy, so I went back to sleep. Either I needed more sleep, or I was dreaming. I woke back up, and things were still the same. I finally got out of bed and fell. I could not walk or see. I called my sister's name to come to our room. I told her I couldn't see or walk. She thought I was playing. I informed her I wasn't playing around.

I usually joke with my siblings but not this time. I asked my sister to run me a bath hoping it would wake me up. I never made it to the bathroom. The water ran over, and water was everywhere. Since our room was across from the bathroom, water was in our room also. I yelled, "China, China. Turn off the water." As I pulled myself up off the floor, it felt like someone grabbed my heart and ripped it out. I screamed for mom. She ran out of her room into ours. I started foaming at the mouth. I was having a seizure. My mother started screaming for my sister to call 911. When the paramedics arrived, I was still seizing, and my pressure was 200/160. They were doing everything they could to save my life. The paramedic told my mother I was pregnant.

From the moment I started to seize, I have no memory of anything. I was told later by my mother about everything that happened. My mother said she continued to argue with the paramedic, guaranteeing her that I was not pregnant. The paramedic responded with, "Ma'am, if we don't take her now, she is going to die." My mother was being told some shocking news. Her 15-year-old daughter was dying and expecting a child at the same time. My mother called my father on the phone. I placed her in a situation because she didn't know what to tell him. She let him know they were taking me to GP Hospital, and he needed to come now. According to my father, he was driving like a speed demon. He drove through traffic lights as he panicked. I know he was confused about what was going on.

As I arrived at the hospital, I continued to have seizures as they prepared me for an emergency C-Section. My blood pressure continued to rise as they placed ice on my body to cool me down. My father arrived at the hospital; that's when my mother broke the news of him becoming a grandfather. In the same sentence, she told him the baby, and I may not make it. If either of us made it, it would be a miracle. God is powerful! He is my strength. He sent guardian angels to watch over me as I was on the table fighting for my life and my unborn child's.

A few days had passed, and I was awake. I woke up next to a beautiful baby boy to my right and my parents to my left. I quickly shut my eyes and closed them tightly. I was thinking, "Lord, I'm still on earth. I'm still going to be punished and placed on the boat." My parents asked me who the father was, but I refused to tell them. My father told me he was not interested in knowing who he was because there was no face that showed up to claim my child. I was taught never to depend on a man for anything. Asking for child support never once came to mind once my father drilled that into my head. My sister told me my father locked himself in the bathroom at home and cried. That hurt me a lot. My siblings weren't told what was going on, so they didn't know why he was crying.

There was a decision to be made. Would I raise my baby or not? I didn't know what to do. I was digging a bigger hole for myself. The sperm donor never wanted me to bring this beautiful life into the world, and I tried to stop this process, but God had the last word, and this child was meant to be here. Even with God saving our lives, I still wanted to know why. Why did God choose to keep us here? I knew I couldn't raise this child without a job or the help of my parents. The decision I finally made was to give my son up for adoption.

I didn't hold my son. I just kept looking at his beautiful light brown eyes. My parents told the nurse to come back. My

22

mother refused to let me give up this innocent soul to someone who may treat him good or maybe bad. This wasn't happening in this family. We all decided I would keep him. I finally held him. The feeling and love were unremarkable and indescribable but the best feeling in the world. My shining angel was 5 pounds and 1 ounce. He was healthy with no issues. I was discharged a few days later to go home with my son. I wasn't sure what the plan was or how I would raise him, but to my surprise, my parents showed me more support than anything.

I was happy that I hadn't experienced any sleepless nights as most new parents do. But I guess I spoke too soon. This child cried his ass off, and I said, "Oh hell no." This boy didn't know who his mother was. I didn't have a problem with giving him love and care. I was used to watching my siblings and babysitting, but this was different. I wasn't getting paid to do this. My mother had to leave nursing school to help me take care of my son. This was a sacrifice my mother made because she cared for and loved me. Even with the disrespect I displayed and the disappointment, she protected me.

The word had got out around the neighborhood that I was home with a baby. Someone told the sperm donor, and apparently, he had been calling my house for a few days, but my father would just answer and hang up once he heard a male's voice asking to speak with me. He finally got in touch with me by phone. Both of my parents were at work, and when I answered the phone, he asked if there was a baby there. I told him yes, it was, and then he let me know he was on the way. I didn't know how I would react to seeing him or what he would say. I couldn't turn back now. I needed to accept whatever words would roll off his tongue or how he would react when he saw our baby.

The donor knocked on the door, and I was scared out of my mind. I opened the door, and he entered. I showed him our son. He held him for a little while, and the way he just stared into his eyes was like he was in deep thought. I could see his passion for our miracle, and I knew he couldn't question much about anything. That was the first and last time he ever held or saw our son until the next ten years. I never revealed to my parents who were responsible for my pregnancy. He didn't want to be revealed anyway.

Adjustment

Weeks had gone by, and it's time for me to return to school to complete the 10th grade. I didn't know who would watch my son. I didn't have any money for daycare. I didn't have any grandmothers here in America like my other friends. I was clueless about everything because I didn't know anything about daycare vouchers or receiving government assistance. My baby was still considered a secret in the African community. I thought this was a joyful situation to share amongst the community. But they were my thoughts only.

My father is Muslim. He was known to brag about what he accepts and does not accept. As his first born, I attended Arabic school on Sundays, which I enjoyed. Not the part of waking up, but the part I was learning to write my name and understand the meaning behind being a Muslim. I felt like there were so many rules in that world. My mother is a Christian who always said if you live under her roof, you must go to church or the mosque you choose, but you must get up and pray.

Some days I went to church as well. I prayed in both the mosque and church. And they both had rules, but those rules have now been broken in my eyes. There was no need to ask one of the old ladies in the Sierra Leone community to watch my child. The fucked-up part was the sperm donors' mother was running a daycare out of her house. I could have asked her to watch him, but I had to be real. This fool did not tell his mother or family anything about having a son. He was engaged and had a new baby two weeks after I had my son. I was 15 years old, and he was 19, and technically that was considered statutory rape. I was inside of a box stuck. I needed to figure this out quickly so I could get back to school.

The time came to decide on what we would do as far as childcare. My parents decided that the best thing would be to send my son to Ghana, West Africa. My mother's sister, Patricia, would take care of him until I completed high school. My parents figured out a way to come up with the money to buy my mother and son a ticket. My mom was going to drop him off at my aunt's. I had to say goodbye for now, but not forever. I would make sure we would be together soon and prove to everyone that I could be a great mother.

He resided in Ghana with my Aunt Patricia for two years until it was time for her to leave Ghana. Once she left Ghana, my mother's oldest sister Gabriela traveled from Sierra Leone to pick him up and bring him back with her to Sierra Leone. This is where she and my grandmother raised him for the next year. It was a crazy situation. The one place I was trying to avoid, my son, ended up there for a year. I wasn't happy at all with the news. This is why I avoided bringing a baby into this world and being unable to provide for him. Now, I wasn't able to see him.

I was returning to school and ready to face whatever came my way. Everyone asked me questions, like, where was I? Or if I had a baby? I heard all kinds of rumors like; I didn't have a baby. Why would anyone make up something like that? I told a different story many times; half of the time, I couldn't remember what I told one person. Overall, those who really knew the truth are who I grew up with in my neighborhood. They knew I did give birth, who the father was, and where I had been. I had to push all of that to the back of my mind, though. I needed to get back to my role and keep up with my image.

I started to mess up even more. My head was twisted and all over the place. I was sneaking out of the house, and I didn't care about any of the rules or regulations my parents set. During this time, my aunt and two cousins were staying with us. A family of five has now turned into eight people living in a 2-bedroom apartment. I had to give up my bed and my room. My family invaded it. Since I love my cousin and we had been together since birth, I liked her being there. It was always us because we were close to age. We're only four months apart but let her tell it; she's a whole year older than me. Now that I knew she was staying with me, there was more fun to have. This was my chance to get my mind off of all this chaos that I was going through. Even with my aunt and cousins living there, I never told them what happened. This was my favorite aunt, but I had to keep my secret in the bag.

My mother helped raise my aunt's children. She was a second mother to them. We were all so close, but when I placed my parents in a tight spot with me having a baby, my parents did not talk to anyone about it. They were hurt when they eventually found out, especially my favorite aunt. But I didn't intend to hurt her or anyone else. Eisha was my favorite cousin, and she loved to have fun like me. We were always at the basketball court and hung out together. She took me to my first concert. We went to see TI. Everyone knows I love that man! We traveled out of town, went to the clubs, and did everything together. She made me feel like I had nothing to worry about in this world. To most, this may sound like two fast-ass girls hanging out. But we weren't fast at all.

Eisha and I go way back! I used to have her sneaking out of the house even when she didn't want to. I would tell her to come, and she would always say she didn't want to or no. I would turn around and threaten her or start yelling. I was a bully towards her. I remember one time I planned on sneaking out. I wanted to go out, but Eisha didn't want to. She told me it wasn't a good night, and we should stay home. Usually, my threats would work but not this time. She didn't move. As much as I wanted her to come, I was going alone. I planned to have a good ass time, and I did. I didn't do anything special outside of being out past my curfew.

In my house, everyone was in bed no later than 11 pm. My parents always had the chain on the door, so the house was on lockdown. I came back in the house thinking everyone was still in bed. I turned the knob quiet as hell and when I opened the door, guess who the hell was sitting in the living room? It was Shaka Zulu and his queen. My father had already called the police to find me. I got caught because my father heard something, and when he went to check around the house, he noticed the chain was off the door. When he went to place the chain back on the door, he saw the unlocked door. He went to check in my room, and I wasn't there. He started questioning my sister and Eisha.

The police officer who came to my house knew who I was, so he told my parents where I was and went to get me. I guess we missed each other, but when I was caught, my father called the officer, and he came back to the house. I went outside to speak with him, and the next thing I know, I was being handcuffed. I didn't get locked up, but I told them I didn't want to return home. I ended up staying at my best friend's house for no more than two days. That was the worst feeling ever. I wasn't eating steak and seafood every day, but I was surviving off of noodles. I had to figure shit out for myself and was staying in a house full of traffic. This was the house I would sneak out to at night to hang out with my friends. The sperm donor found out I was there, and I wanted to go home. In less than 48 hours, I was begging my father to let me come home. I didn't have to beg my father; he wanted me to come back. That was all he had to say because I was gone. This was one of those moments when I was thankful for what I had. I knew I needed to cherish my life; it wasn't that bad.

One day I was at home with my family. Not sure what triggered me this day, but my mother and I had gotten into a big altercation. Rage and hate towards my mother came out as I told her that my son should not have gone to Africa and they weren't going to allow me to see him again. I was convinced there were other resources to use. My mother said one word, and I blacked out. Nothing she was saying to me I heard. I started to swing, and I ended up fighting my mother. My aunt broke the fight up. My mother is 5'3" and the woman who sacrificed her world for mines. I knew I was going to hell for putting my hands on my mother. Well, that is according to the bible. Don't get it twisted because she whipped my ass and made me remember who the hell I was dealing with.

A lot of people would ask, why was I out of control and so angry? I could only think about my son and the stupid choices I made. I was not learning from my mistakes. I continued to sleep with the enemy. All that was being told to me, being whispered, or being placed in my head was not true. My parents meant good behind what they did when they sent my son to Africa. The resources were available, but they may not have worked for me. My parents never said I wasn't going to get him back. They said I needed to finish school on time.

It was the summer of 2003, and I was headed to the 11th grade. I was 17 years old and working at a fast-food restaurant. It was my first job. There was money to be made, but it also kept me busy. I had goals I was working towards. Let me be clear I was always a go-getter; nothing or no one can get in my way. I worked as much as I could.

Sometimes I made bad decisions. The sperm donor never acknowledged my son. Even with him not helping me with my son and telling me he's engaged, I continued to sleep with him. He was treating me like a hoe, and I let him. I figured if I continued to give him my body, he would come around, and eventually, when my son came home; he would be there for him as a father. I was hoping my son would come home early. If he does, he can tell his family, and I can finally let my family know who the father of my child is. Because of my mission, I think I had more sex that year than ever. There was no progress with the donor, and my mission had failed.

That same year I met Ricardo. Ricardo was chilled and always laid back with shades on. It looked like he always had shades on because he wore glasses. Whenever the sun was out, his glasses would turn into sunglasses. Ricardo was from around my way but lived on the other side of me. We clicked, and he would give me a ride home from school sometimes. We balanced each other's energy. I started to become close with him like I was with Calvin and Zion. Ricardo was different. I never thought we would get that close.

My parents took care of my son while he was in Africa. They never asked me for a dime, even if I offered anything. My Aunt Patricia had one son and took care of my little cousin. This showed me she had a big and caring heart. It takes a special person to add another child to your family. This was a major sacrifice to me. It takes a village to raise kids, and with the team I had behind me, I was grateful. I gave my parents a hard time, but to be honest, no one understood me or understood exactly what I was going through. I had a baby at 15, I had to keep secrets, built-up rage, nowhere to turn, and with all of this, I had to satisfy my parents. I was a lot to handle, and that resulted in disappointing them.

I always had big dreams. I never thought of myself as anything less. I always spoke my dreams into the atmosphere. My dream was to become a Pediatric Nurse and go to the Air force. As much as I wanted to join the Air Force, I didn't like the discipline. As I thought about the long boot camp training, someone in your face yelling and waking up at crazy hours was bogus to me. My dreams then turned into bringing my son home and providing him with everything. We needed to catch up on everything I had missed and providing him with all he needed. I only had a year to get it together and prepare for my shining angel to come home.

Certain parts of my life were all over the place. Joshua came back into the picture. There was history between us, but he never knew I was pregnant. He later found out I had given birth. He was calling me nonstop. When he got a hold of me, I told him I had been in the hospital because of my blood pressure and had to be placed on ice. We met in person some months later, once my son had been taken to Africa. He probably did not believe me, but it was the truth, and I didn't need to explain myself any further. It may seem messed up in some people's eyes, but we dated each other in the past. Plus, I was still dealing with the sperm donor, so we went our separate ways. I was long gone and so caught up with someone that didn't want me.

Senior year had arrived. I made it, and this was the year my parents promised me my son would come home. It was a long road, but I was going to get what I wanted. I know I wasn't the best daughter to my parents and a great example for my siblings, but I had my own mind. No one was going to control me unless they understood me.

Joshua and I got back together again. We were going to each other's prom. I was working at the time, so I was able to pay for everything myself. I never asked my parents to do anything for me during my senior year. They did enough by taking care of my son. I had to get two dresses made. My prom was a big deal; therefore, I wanted to do it big. I was not going to the store and buy a dress; I wanted my dress to be made.

On the day of my prom, I needed a ride to the metro. I didn't plan to work because I had so much to do in such little time. In my mind, there was only one person to give me a ride. I called the sperm donor. He came to pick me up. We headed straight to his house and did what we did. I kept asking myself when I was going to set standards for myself. I was still a little girl in his eyes that could easily be taken advantage of. I keep falling for him as if he's going to be around when my son comes home. This was the day when everything finally clicked in my head. He was useless and not worth it. It was no longer about how I felt, and I needed to stop making excuses for his actions. He was a boy in a man's body. I always hoped he would admit his wrongdoings and grow up. That was the last day I had sex with him. I had finally realized my worth.

My mother was getting ready to go to Sierra Leone to get my son. She was taking my sister and brother on vacation. It was 2005, and so much had happened. There's a saying, "Keep your friends close and your enemies closer." This is the most accurate saying I had ever heard. When I had my son, my parents lost friends and family because they chose not to tell anyone. No one said anything to my parents about it; they were just whispering. None of that surprised me because that's how the African community is. They are always judging someone, but the whole time their lives are more complicated than anyone else's. Even with their messed-up life, they didn't care. Like anyone else, they swept their mess under the rug.

My heritage is very prideful and extraordinarily strong, and I will do anything to protect my family. Family is just as bad as outsiders. When my son was in Ghana, one of my aunts on my father's side was transitioning to America, but she told everyone I had a baby by a white man. It sounds ridiculous, but it was all about image, and they liked congosa, which means gossip. I was tired of hiding my precious jewel.

New Beginning

I graduated high school, and I was still working at a fast-food restaurant. I mentioned before I wanted to go into the Air Force and become a Pediatric Nurse, but I also wanted to attend the University of Maryland like my father. My plans changed because I didn't have the grades. I ended up going to Prince Georges County Community College. Before I started college, I confided in my mother that I wanted to get into the nursing program to become a licensed practical nurse. After that, I would go to the University to get my bachelor's in nursing. My mother had other plans. Instead, she told me what I was going to do. She placed me in a certified nursing assistant class while taking regular courses to get into the nursing program at Prince Georges Community College.

My mother always told me that there was no real money to be made working in retail. I had financial aid for school, worked at the daycare on campus, was an assistant manager at Family Dollar, and was still looking for a job in the field as a Certified Nursing Assistant. Everything felt good to me. I was working hard, taking care of my son, had a car, and was not dependent on anyone. Things were coming together for me, especially when, at one point, everything and everyone was against me. Life was finally turning around, at least that's what I thought.

The moment that I have been waiting for was finally here. It was as if I had been pregnant all over again, but this time, I was pregnant for three years. I felt like I was about to go into labor with a splash of adrenaline rushing through my blood. I was ecstatic and anxious. What was I going to say to my three-year-old son? I hadn't seen him since he was six weeks old. There were so many thoughts running through my mind. Should I apologize to him? Would he remember me? Will he call me mommy?

The Journey of the Unbreakable Warrior

My father and I went to the airport to meet my mother, siblings, and son. I wasn't able to sit still in the car. I watched the time go by with every second and minute. We finally arrived at the airport, and I was a nervous wreck waiting for them to get off the plane. I was thinking about how I would react when I saw him. I saw my mother and my sister, but behind is trailing my brother and my shining angel. He was holding tight to my brother's hands. I could tell he didn't want to let him go. He looked at me but with a look like, "who are you?" My son didn't run to me, he didn't call me mommy, and he had no idea who I was. None of that mattered. I was happy he was here because I was able to see and touch him.

My wish had finally come true. I could touch, smell, and see my beautiful son. He had a big head but the cutest lips, fat cheeks, and a swag of a millionaire at three years old. My son did not like me. He only went to my brother and my mother, who he called Mama. He couldn't speak English, so our communication was not on point, but I understood him because my parents spoke Creo to us as children, but we did not speak it back. I knew that would not last long because all I spoke was English, so he would have to adapt, especially when he started school.

My son is back home, and Joshua and I were in a relationship again. Joshua immediately stepped up to be a father to my son. I never asked him to take the role of being a father or even brought up what he would do once he got home. He chose the role, and I respected his decision. In my mind, I was still a single parent who had responsibilities and a little person looking up to me. I would always carry the title of being an independent black woman who would never depend on a man.

At 19-years-old, I picked up the responsibilities of a mother, and I will not lie to you; it was hard in the beginning because I had to earn my son's trust. But I did that, and we were close. I introduced Joshua to my son as Daddy because Joshua wished for him to be called that. It felt funny at first, but I can see the love that this man had for him, and he was not biologically his. I guess when you love someone, whatever they come with, you except. Joshua's family also welcomed my prince with open arms and as their own. You would have never thought that he was not a part of them. It was great to know that I had that support and did not even think twice about reaching out to the sperm donor.

The sperm donor did not want to be a father or take responsibility anyway; I just made it easier for him. I was maxed out of options to keep trying. Even though there were other ways like child support, I couldn't do it. I never believed in the court system. I didn't care if it is one dollar or a hundred dollars; it wasn't enough for my son. I wasn't looking for a financial come-up; I wanted a man to be a father to my son. I had my little family, and I was fine with that. If he wanted to be a father, he would have. I was going to protect my son at all cause. I wasn't going to send him somewhere where he was unwanted.

If there was one thing about me, I kept my son clean. I took good care of him. I paid for his daycare, bought his clothes and shoes. I spoiled my child. It wasn't to replace the time that I missed, but it was genuine love and the time I could give him. I started working at an assisted living home, making $10.00 an hour. It wasn't a lot of money, but it was more than $6.75 during that time. It wasn't a lot at the assistant living home, but I was still working at the daycare center on campus, doing retail, and getting a refund check from school. I considered this to be an okay income to take care of my shining star and myself.

I said it takes support and a village to raise children. I had the support and a village that consisted of Zion and Calvin.

Calvin spoiled my son from birthday parties to anything he wanted. He was the uncle that could get him the gadget or pair of shoes that no one had. Because of Calvin, my son had the new releases before anyone else. Of course, once Eisha was aware of him being here or even me being a mother, she wasted no time being the best aunt that she could be. She was always someone I could depend on for anything. Honestly, I felt like I depended on her a little too much. But my team was built solid.

When my son turned five years old, he was such a big boy, smart, and loved Lil Wayne's song, Fireman. Every time that song came on, he was in front of that TV dancing. He wasn't doing just any kind of dancing; he was cool and smooth with it as he wore a hat on his head. He always said he wanted to be a firefighter. By the time he turned five, he didn't speak Creo, there was no accent, and he called me mommy and Joshua, daddy.

We were all living together. Then, something happened. I don't know what you would call it, but it wasn't the right time. I was pregnant with Joshua's baby. It would make sense to keep the baby because of everything I went through with my first pregnancy. No! Sorry, it wasn't a good time. Neither of us was ready. I still needed to bond with my son. I was in school and financially not stable. An abortion it was. This was one of the most hurtful and devastating feelings in the world. There was a little seed growing inside of me that didn't ask to be created. It was a hard decision but the right one.

The day was scheduled for me to get an abortion, and there were protesters outside of the building. What in the hell was going on? Maybe it was a sign or God telling me to turn around. I sat in the car for a little to think, and I tell you I was thinking hard as hell, but I had to go through with it. I needed to prove that I can be a great mother to my first child and accomplish what I already started. We have a forgiving God, and I asked for forgiveness. After the abortion was done, my mother and Joshua's mother were both aware of this pregnancy; this was no secret. My mother wanted me to get an abortion. She felt like this was not the right time, and I needed to finish school. Unlike Joshua's mother, when it was done, she gave me the cold shoulder. I mean, this lady was nonchalant and rolling her eyes while she smoked her cigarette. I paid her no mind. I knew what was best for me, and this was a decision that Joshua and I made together.

Jump

A few years after I graduated from high school, my parents decided to move to Bowie, Maryland. Honestly, they did not want my siblings to end up at the same school and situation I was in. I was already giving them a run for their money. Things were going great, but as I said, I always had heavy thoughts on my mind. When we moved to our new house, my parents wanted us to have our own space. It was so beautiful. It was a 3-level townhouse. When you entered to the right, there was an open space and a kitchen with a wide window. Next to the kitchen was the dining room. Going further in, there was the living room. To get to it, you had to go down three steps with a deck. We had a big basement which was pretty much my space because no one came downstairs.

I have two siblings, my sister China and my brother Ali. Ali had his own room even though he shared it with my son. Ali and my son shared a room; my son always slept with me. China and I had to share a room. I wasn't happy at all. Even though I had my son home and things were great, I still had this nonchalant and aggressive attitude. I loved my siblings and would do anything for them, but they could be annoying at times. China and I did not have a relationship at the time. I guess she looked more at my flaws than my heart. Ali, he went with the flow of things; whatever he saw is how he felt. He went with the energy that my parents gave when they called me out on my behavior.

I did not make it any better because I lashed out at him and didn't mean to. One day my brother annoyed me so bad that we fought. We physically fought because he had to put his two cents in a conversation that had nothing to do with him. As we were arguing, I attacked him and threw the dining room chair at him. A ticking time bomb that had just exploded on her brother for no reason. There were times when the bomb should have gone off, like when I was around the donor. But it didn't.

Time and years have passed. I am now in Chapter 23, and at this point, Joshua and I live together, and my shining Star is seven years old. We were in a happy place, or should I say a better space. We were happy but don't get it twisted because there were issues. Joshua was one sneaky individual. He was never the type to just get it like I was, and he always thought he was a step ahead, but I was three steps forward.

Every person has flaws. I had set goals and was working hard to provide for my child and me. I worked doubles as a Certified Medicine Technician. I was working two jobs. I loved Joshua for his laughs, looks, and personality, but we were not on the same page as far as goals. That didn't mean I had to give up on him. I had to give him a chance. There was no way I could give up on a man who has accepted my son as his own. Joshua not setting goals was something minor. I couldn't let it bother me. I couldn't fix him. My job was to let him know what I expected and see what happened from there.

Everyone thought the brothers I gained along the way were my biological brothers. I could make one phone call with my boy's problems, and they would be there. At this age, the three amigos were going through a withdrawal. I was pulling closer to Ricardo. Not intentionally. I loved my brothers. It was just a time in my life where I felt like Ricardo was there more than Calvin and Zion. You know how they say people come into your life for a season. Our seasons were changing. There was no love lost or forgotten. I had no idea what was ahead of us.

While working at the assisted living home, I became good friends with a girl named Crystal. We would hang out and go to reggae parties most of the time. One night when we were going out, I was driving a 2006 Hyundai Elantra. My mother helped me purchase this car. When we bought the vehicle at a used car dealership, we were given temporary Georgia tags when it was purchased. We were told after 30 days, my Maryland hard tags would arrive, and I could come to pick them up from him. Those 30 days turned into 60 days until the night Crystal and I was going out. The plan was for her to do my hair, get dressed, and go to the reggae club.

My car was parked in front of her house on a one-way street. In less than 30 seconds of getting into the car, a police officer pulled behind me. He knocked on the window and asked me for my documents. I asked him why he stopped, and I didn't pull out of the parking spot yet. He refused to tell me anything until I gave him my license and registration. I wasn't worried about anything because my paperwork was good. Even though my stuff was good, I was nervous. This was the first time the police stopped me. I was shaking as if I had Parkinson's. I wasn't moving fast enough for him, so he reached into my car to grab my purse. He dumbed everything out into my lap so he could get my license. My reflex caused my fist to go flying to the officer's face. My window was halfway down, so he proceeded to open my door. I was fighting back.

Backup arrived, and he was able to get me out of the car. He pushed me up against the car, and he spread my legs. As he was kicking my feet out to spread them, I started to urinate on him. I was nervous, and I had to use the bathroom, so I peed. He wasn't happy by the look on his face. I wasn't thinking. I was defending and protecting myself. From the time he approached my car, I knew he was up to no good. I was placed in the back of his car, cursing and talking trash the whole time. I told him I was going to spit on him and some other things. This officer wasn't white; he was black. The other officers drove my car away. I knew what they did wasn't right. They were supposed to call a tow truck to transport my car to the impound. I know the procedures. I knew how they were handling things, and something wasn't right. I was eventually told my tags were illegal. How was I supposed to know that? My mother and I thought they were a legit dealer. I was transported to Hyattsville Jail, and when we arrived, he stopped instantly. My first thought was he would rape or kill me. We weren't in the woods or a closed area.

We were at the station in the back where they take you for processing. He began to erase the feed on the camera. His ass was a dirty cop. He then got out of the car to get me out of the back seat and took me to the station. Of course, I had to get processed. They put me in an orange jumpsuit because I was wet and smelling like urine. I got all dolled up only for me to end up in jail. I spoke to a female officer while I was waiting to see the commissioner. I explained to her what took place. She told me the same officer who brought me in had many complaints against him, and even if I went above to report him, it was going to be very tough. I did not even know what would happen to me, whether I would serve time for resisting arrest or what. Prayers were real.

My name was called to speak with the commissioner. I started shaking again as I stood in front of the commissioner. I was given PBJ, which means Probation Before Judgement. I was able to go home but still had to go to court. I don't know how that was the only charge I received, but I didn't ask any questions. I did go to court, and the officer who arrested me showed up. I explained to the judge exactly what and how I bought my vehicle. I wanted to go deeper about the officer's action, but at the moment, all I could remember is what the female officer had told me. I was thankful that I only received PBJ. As far as the dealer who I bought my car from, his ass disappeared. He packed up shop and left. I could not do anything with my car because I had no title. I wasn't the only one this dealer did this to. Overall, everything worked out in my favor.

After all that chaos, I found out I was expecting! Yes, I was pregnant! We were finally receiving some good news. I was four weeks along, and I felt like this was going to be a long pregnancy. This time around, we decided to keep the baby. We had no reason not to do so. We were mature adults that placed ourselves in a situation. Plus, this was going to be Joshua's first biological child. This was a happy moment for both of us. And now it is time to tell the parents. I was no longer a 15-year-old, and I didn't have to keep this big secret. I wasn't depressed, and there was no need to overdose. I was now mature, and I knew I could do this. I was capable of being a mother of two. I was in a stable relationship, even though we had issues, but what relationship didn't. The only thing I knew was I had to prepare myself to tell my parents I was pregnant. I needed to tell my parents separately.

While I was preparing myself to tell my parents, my mother got to me first. She told me my father found my Kaiser papers. It didn't even cross my mind that my health insurance was under my father's name, and all of my papers were going to my parent's house. My mother asked me what I would do, and I told her that I would keep the child. She agreed and said my job now was to go and talk to my father. Now I had to prepare for the big dogs. I am about to have a sit-down with Shaka Zulu. I called my father to ask which day would work for him for me to come over so that we can talk. He told me whenever I was ready in the evening. Whatever day I was choosing, I had to suck it up. The day came for me to sit down with my father, and I was nervous, but it just rolled off my tongue. "Well, daddy, you already know as you read my Kaiser paper that I am pregnant."

My Father asked if it was Joshua's baby. I was like, duh, who else, baby would it be? Of course, I knew it was part of the process of him asking questions. After that question, my father said, "Okay, well, we have known Joshua for years now since you guys were younger. This is who we know for our grandson's father. So, we support you in your decision, and we will be there for you as our daughter." I was shocked by everything he said. Did I hear him correctly? For the first time in my life, I felt like I could tell my parents anything at this point. They supported me through my decision. Little did I know I would need my parent's support on this journey for sure.

Nine months seemed so far down the road. I ended up being a high-risk patient. I always believed when I was giving birth to my son, I died. I say I returned from the dead. I had eclampsia during that pregnancy, so they labeled me as a high risk this time around. I had to go to the doctor for a checkup every two weeks to make sure that the baby and I were okay. Even with being high risk, this pregnancy felt great. I worked, took care of the home, and was just glowing even through the high blood pressure experience. I guess you can say it was a happy weight, but I looked good.

My blood type is O negative, so I had to go through some tests and drink that drink that doesn't taste very pleasant. Even with me going through all these tests and going to the doctor every two weeks, it didn't bother me. I finally had the experience of going to get a check-up and taking prenatal pills. This, to me, was my first pregnancy, even though it was not. But I am going through everything I should have gone through with my son.

It was time for us to find out what we were having. I already knew without any doctor telling me, just like I knew with my son. I was having a girl. During the ultrasound, I was so calm but excited just for those words to roll off her tongue, "You're having a girl." Joshua and I were happy. The feeling of joy when you feel like everything is complete, but this was just the beginning.

The day my baby girl was to enter the world, she decided she needed a grand entrance. And of course, she gave one. In April 2008, my mother was out of the country. That wasn't the plan, but she scheduled her trip around the time I was supposed to deliver. I kept getting these sharp pains in the middle of the night but not consistently, but those pains were no joke. As the night went on, I kept getting these pains, so I decided to call the 24-hour nurse line. They told me to take a cold shower and go for a walk. What the hell kind of advice was that to give me? All of this was new to me. They were the experts, so I did what they told me. Nothing was working for me at all. I called my father, who had no clue either but to say call 911. I ended up calling Joshua's mother because both of our cars were down, and the rental that we had needed to be returned a few days before my due date. When I called his mother, I told her that I have an appointment in the morning, and I have been in pain. I told her I thought I was going into labor. First off, you will not believe what this lady said, "Girl, you not going into labor, but I will be there in the morning."

The next morning arrived, and I thought I was going to Kaiser. This lady was going to show houses. Yes! Houses! What the fuck? I was so furious that smoke was coming out of every part of me. I could barely sit in the chair. It felt like I had to take a shit. I didn't expect labor to make me feel like that. It was the most uncomfortable feeling ever. I needed someone to get me out of that car. This lady thought it was a joke. When she finally finished showing her house, and she dropped me off at Kaiser. When I got there, they did the ultrasound and came to find out my baby was under stress, and my blood pressure was sky high along with my baby's heart rate dropping. All of this could have been avoided, but there was no time for the should've, could've, would've.

Joshua was called, and apparently, the apple does not fall too far from the tree. I have never been so scared to ride in the car with this fool. His ass couldn't see or drive already, but he got me to the hospital as fast as he could. They had to do an emergency c section for her to come out because I would not be able to push her out. I did want to have that experience, but I could not. The only thing that mattered to me was for me to be able to have a safe delivery.

My princess made her entrance. She was so beautiful with a head full of hair. I had my Princess and Prince. Going through that pregnancy was a different feeling and experience for me. It was like I was a first-time mother when technically I was. After having my daughter, I started experiencing high blood pressure and frequent migraines. Even though I already had that at 15 years old, this had to be controlled with medication.

Ever since I was a baby, I always had a skin rash off and on. It would come and go with the treatment of different creams. Of course, the first thing that they say is that it was eczema, and as I got older, they said psoriasis. My parents constantly took me to a specialist. When I was five years old, in 1991, my father went to Sierra Leone for my grandfather's funeral. At the time, my mother could not drive, so they decided to take me to New Jersey so that my aunt could help take care of me while my father traveled and my mother worked. My father received a disturbing phone call from my uncle stating that I was in bad condition and needed to get me from my aunt's house. When my father arrived from Sierra Leone, he drove to New Jersey to pick me up. When he saw me, he asked what happened. He wanted to know if I had an allergic reaction to something. My aunt told him that I didn't have anything that would give me an allergic reaction and that nothing happened. She assured my father that it was just my Eczema. My parents then drove me back to Maryland and rushed me to Children's Hospital. This has been an ongoing process, and when I became older, it did not get any better. My breakouts began to leave scars, and I started having more flare-ups. Little did I know that at 23 years old, I would be diagnosed with Lupus.

I always felt fatigued, had skin breakouts and migraines. One day I made a doctor's appointment, and I had been to so many doctors, and this one was no different. That's what I thought. When I went to my appointment, it was this small office, and I thought it was ghetto. Well, I am hood, but I am bougie hood when I need to be. I was sitting in this doctor's office, and the wait was forever, but I waited because I just was tired of feeling this way and breaking out. After being called to the back, he asked me several questions about my history. He was also looking at my skin outbreak. This rash, in particular, was different. I had a rash that was formed like a butterfly across my nose. Not even 5 minutes into the exam, he asked the tech to take my blood work. He was going to run some tests, and that was it. Within the next 48 hours, I received a phone call stating that he wanted me to come back to his office to read my results and he needed to see me immediately. I wanted to know why the doctor needed me to come back in. Did I have something? Was it that bad that he couldn't tell me over the phone? I was going to go anyway, but I needed to call my parents.

My mother went with me to my appointment, and the doctor explained that he did a few tests, and my results came back that I have SLE. The expression on my face was what in the hell was SLE. If this nigga gave me an SLE, I am fitting to kill him. I told him I never had an STD. He repeated himself and let me know it was SLE, not an STD. He needed to speak words I could understand.

"You have Lupus! It is called Systemic Lupus Erythematosus and Discoid Lupus which is DLE," my doctor explained. So, the overall diagnosis was SLE/DLE Stage 3 Kidney Nephritis.

I was lost, and I did not understand the language and was confused. The doctor then explained what the disease is and said that it was 100% in my DNA, and I had a lot of protein in my urine, which my kidneys were being attacked, and we had to take action right away. I felt so numb, and not knowing what the cause of this did not make it any better. The Lupus caused my flare-ups with my rash, but who would have thought that.

The doctor then referred me to a Nephrologist in Greenbelt, Maryland. The Nephrologist was expecting me, so I went to his office right away. He ran his test and said I needed to go to Holy Cross Hospital to do a procedure on my kidneys, a biopsy, to test it to see what needed to be done. This was just way too much for me at this point. I was agitated. I couldn't show how I felt because I had to be strong. We scheduled a time and date. The time had come for me to get the biopsy done. Once that was done, that test came back and showed that I had a mild case which I was diagnosed with stage 3 Kidney Nephritis. The amount of protein shown in my urine was a lot, but action was taken right away when it was caught. My whole life started to change right before my eyes. But it did not stop me from being me.

I was placed on different medications to control my blood pressure, heart rate, and kidneys. It was a lot to control. I never thought this could happen to me; at 23-years-old I refused to allow this to stop me. I was not too fond of the suspense feeling that I had of not knowing if I would wake up the next morning. That was something I never imagined. We are all born to die, but I wouldn't wish this on my worst enemy. Honestly, if I didn't have children to live for, I could care less. I felt like I was being penalized for everything I had done. I knew I was a sinner, but who wasn't. I was the first one in my family to have this disease in my body. How would anyone know that it was hereditary? My family wasn't from this country. There was no way I could go down my family line to find out where it came from. The best way to handle what I was experiencing was to live and not think of what I was going through.

I was going through pain, and I received treatment through IV every two weeks for 4 hours. This disease needed to be taken seriously. With all I had going on, you would think I would begin to eat right, exercise, and educate myself more on this disease. I was possibly opening the door for new diseases. I was being told not to eat this or that and exercise. I was being asked questions, like do you know that Lupus can do this or that? I couldn't answer any of the questions right away. I was living in the moment and not thinking about the future that would affect me down the line. It was taking a toll on me, but I never showed it. I felt like I was in a world of destruction and the only way to defeat this battle was to brush it off and not show any weakness. Instead of showing weakness, the ticking time bomb was active again.

I was filled with anger even before I was diagnosed with Lupus or the Tolosa Hunt Syndrome episode. I dealt with this by fighting, and the bad part was, I held it all in. That was dangerous. Can you imagine having so much built inside that needed to come out, and when you let it out, someone innocent or has nothing to do with how you feel gets the raft? But no one understood me or knew how I felt, so I thought. My cousin Eisha knew me well and can read me like a book.

As time went on, I did not experience any major changes but keeping up with medication was a new thing. It didn't truly sink in that I was diagnosed with something or that I had something in my body, yet alone if I do not take care of myself, I can die from it.

Roller Coaster

I loved to have fun, party, and look good. But most importantly, being a mother to my two children. I had to live for them and be able to see them grow into intelligent and successful young men and women. I was known for throwing parties, and they were always fun. Ms. Unpredictable is what I called myself at this time of my life. I had so many parties I was building my own entertainment company, Unpredictable Entertainment.

Chapter 24 was quite interesting. At the time, I was working as a transporter at Walter Reed Hospital. This day I left for work from Eisha's house, and it was raining. My car was giving me trouble, but that was not stopping me from going to make money. While on the beltway, my car started smoking and broke down on the side of the road. This was not a good time for my car to break down. It wasn't all about missing work but my tags. I needed to renew my tags, but I did not do it once they expired, so I decided to use a photocopy of someone else tags. These were not black and white. They were colored copied on white paper with a clear cover to protect them. It sounds insane, but I got away with it until this day.

A police officer pulled behind me to assist or ask did I need help. This occurred at 4 am so it was still dark outside. The first time he approached my window, he asked why I was pulled over, and I explained my vehicle broke down and wouldn't start. You can hear the cracking in my voice. He then asked for my license and registration. This police officer was about to get some expired documentation or a sob ass story. I gave him my driver's license and told him I misplaced my registration. He went back to his vehicle, and a few minutes later, a second police car arrived. Before he could approach my window the second time, I gave Eisha a call to tell her to let my job know I will not be able to make it. She needed to get to me right away because I knew I was going to jail.

When he returned, he said, "Do you know that your license is suspended, and where did you get your tags? Is that a photocopy?" There was no point in lying. I was going down telling the truth. I was caught. I said, "Yes, it is a copy, and no, I was not aware of my license being suspended." Well, I gave half the truth and a lie. Eisha pulled up and asked what station I was being transported to. I was already in cuffs and placed in the backseat of the police car. She followed us, and when I arrived at the station, I was the laughingstock that day.

They all wanted to know how I got away with this. I said that was the only way I could get back and forth to work. I did not stay in holding for long. I was released about three hours later. I didn't mind being the laughingstock if that kept me out of jail. I knew that my license was suspended, but I had no choice now but to get everything registered with the state, or it was going to affect my money. You already know I didn't learn my lesson, but life must go on.

It took three other times before I finally got it. The next time wasn't because of traffic, but it was for love. Joshua and I decided to go to Annapolis Mall one day, and I was driving. While driving on route 50, Joshua decided to smoke his blunt in my car. I spotted the police officer miles away behind me and started to push the petal to the metal. I mean, I was going at least 67 miles at first until I spotted them and went 90. I had an eye for the police, so I knew what kind of car they were in undercover and where they hid. The police officer caught up to us and ended up pulling me over. He did not pull me over because he knew we had weed in the car; it was because I was speeding. Before he could pull me over, I told Joshua to get rid of it. He decides to put it in the soda can.

The police asked for my license and registration but then started to search the car. I guess he smelled the marijuana. He proceeded to grab the soda can and emptied it on the side of the road. When he did, he found the wet blunt and asked who it was. I was quiet at first because I thought Joshua would claim that it was his. But he did not do so. I guess I shouldn't have expected that he would speak up. He was already caught up in his dumb madness, but this was his fall as well. I said it was mine because I didn't smoke, and I had no charges. What was I thinking? I was a ride-or-die chick.

At that time, I was not thinking, but I was loyal. I was transported to Anne Arundel Jail and was placed on a bond for $500. I was wondering if he was going to come through for me as I did for him. It was the wrong time to think about all of that. But he did, and I was later released. When I went to court for this case, the charges were dropped. I think the judge knew that I just agreed to the charges.

After all the foolishness and wild shenanigans, I needed to celebrate hard. I am that person whose birthday is a holiday. You better recognize and observe my day. I love to have parties and fun. I was having a party at Half Note Lounge for my 24th Birthday. I know it was more of an older crowd, but Ricardo's mother had connections. I love to show off, party and be the center of attention when it is my time to shine, and it is about me. The night of my party we were having a great time. All of my friends were there. I was looking like the star that I am. I mean, what can I say? I looked good, and we were drinking and having a great time. Until I had a surprise, unexpected guest. The sperm donor showed up. Yes, I said the sperm donor. This fool was not invited, so I didn't understand why he was there. He tells me how much it has been eating him up that he has not been in our son's life. This was not the right time to talk, and nothing was processing because I was enjoying my birthday party. I snuck out of my party to go to the front entrance. I couldn't talk to him while Joshua was there. This was not the right approach or the right time.

Afterward, I started to think very heavily about what he came to talk to me about, which was my son. All I wanted was for him to be a father to my prince. I reached out to him for us to meet. He was a tattoo artist at this time, so I told him that I wanted to get a tattoo, and I wanted to pierce my son's ears. We met over at my friend Eskay's house for it to be done because I felt like that was the only way we could talk or for me to have his attention. Plus, this was a good place for him to see my son.

I always knew that nothing held a man's attention. Not even a kid. If he does not want his attention to be held, it will not. You cannot force anyone to do anything they do not want to do. Especially taking care of a child or be a father to him. The thoughts and feelings of what to do or doing the right thing were so tormenting and had me distraught. I was ignoring all of the red flags that were placed in front of me. We all ignore the signs. That is exactly what I was doing at this point. It was no longer about me; this was about my son.

While I was getting my tattoo done, we did not even talk about my son. All he was saying about wanting to be there, it has been eating him up, or whatever else he had on his mind when he approached me, he didn't mention any of it. Overall, it was all false advertisement. After my tattoo was finished, he pierced my son's ears, but I never introduced him as anything. All I said to my son was, "Come sit and down to get your ear pierced." How can I introduce a man to my shining star that had no interest? The funny thing is, later, I found out that Eskay and her mother caught the sperm donor standing outside, watching my son while he was playing football with his friend. I mean, the man stood out there for a while, just observing him and watching his every move. What was going on in his mind? How did he feel? I guess I would never know.

Even after pushing myself to be back around this man who had no respect for me, degraded me, and looked at me as though I was just this young dumb girl, he did not budge to make a move to even say out of his mouth, "That's my son" or "How is he doing?" What could I do at this point? I started hanging back around him to see if I could get him around my son or do for him. Of course, it came with a price. I started to sleep with the enemy again. After all the things I have been through mentally, I turned around and slept with this man. There was a cookout that my friends and I put together, and I road with him to the event. If I were to show up with him there, everyone would be surprised or looking at me with crazy eyes. Fuck it. It wasn't about what they thought. I knew why I was dealing with him. And the crazy part is Joshua and I were still together. I was just sneaking around at this point and cheating.

When we got to the cookout, my cousin Eisha was there, and she asked me what the hell was he doing there? She wanted to know what I was doing. Eisha was very protective over me and would not have anyone around my son, even if it is his father or not. I didn't listen to her. I had to see if I could convince him to at least start being around for the sake of my son. We left the cookout, and when he was dropping me off, I asked him to buy my son a pair of shoes. It was like pulling teeth to ask this man anything. It was just a hundred dollars, and it felt like I was asking him for a thousand. I did not get the money right away, but he gave me a hundred dollars to buy my son shoes later. My son was 10-years old at the time, which is the only thing that this man, who is his father, gave or has done for him financially. My father told me never to ask this man for anything or depend on any man, but I went back on my promise and my word. This was the sacrifice I made just for a hundred dollars, and he still wasn't a father to his son.

Ms. Unpredictable

I always wanted to plan and celebrate big for my 25th birthday. And that is what I did. I am Ms. Unpredictable, and it would not be me if I didn't celebrate. But that year, I was going all out. I decided to have a masquerade ball at Plaza 23. This was going to be the party of the year. My favorite color is pink, and I love lace. My dress had to be custom-made. Everything had to be right and exactly how I wanted. It was a short powder pink lace with lavender silk trimming underneath for the bottom and top dress. With 6-inch guess powder pink and lavender heels. My hair was in a blunt-cut bob, and everything was on point from head to toe. I looked like a million bucks. I decided to do flyers so that I could sell tickets. On the flyer, it was a childhood friend who moved from Maryland to Atlanta to pursue his music career and me. At the time, he was making beats for a few artists down there. I placed him as a special guest on my flyer.

I had everyone selling tickets to promote this extravaganza. I knew people would purchase because I always had a good turn out and we always had a ball. What I didn't know was my party would have 200 guests or maybe more. The night of the party, people were still paying at the door. Eisha oversaw the decorations, and it was set up beautifully. It was filled with colorful balloons, and we had our VIP Section, which I never got a chance to even sit down in. Everyone was dressed up so nicely with their mask on. It took me by surprise that no one came underdressed.

The picture booth was always full, and drinks were over the limit. But there was a thief somewhere. I wasn't sure who, but money started to disappear. It was my birthday party, and I could not have fun and guard the door. A good friend did sit at the door for me and collect money initially, but I trusted her. I had to have someone else there so she can at least enjoy herself, and from there, money started disappearing. The music was good to a certain point. Then Eisha had to step in for the music to be changed. You know music is what gets the party going. Well, it had to be at least 45 minutes till the party came to an end. Eisha and the DJ started to exchange words, and my party started to die. The next thing I know, I saw a chair fly somewhere, and a big fight broke out. People were getting pushed, and so did I. I found myself on the floor as well.

Someone had a gun, and for me to have security at the front door, they sure did not do a good job of checking. It is always that one person to act stupid. A misunderstanding occurred, and they took it a step further, wanting to kill. No one was hurt, or no gun shots were fired, but I learned a lesson. In the future, I would not have an open invitation to the public. Overall, my party was a success as usual. I still had a good time, and it was memorable with the bad and good in the end. I can say I had a masquerade ball for my 25th birthday, and we had a ball. On the other hand, I can also say I remember when a fight broke out and police were called because it got out of control.

This same year Eskay and I threw our first annual Luau party. For it to be our first event together, the turnout was unbelievable. You could hear the music from the main road before getting to the street. We had a picture booth, tiki bar, DJ, and anything you can think of; we had it. You saw people walking a distance just to come to the party. It looked as though we were throwing a block party. This was the extravaganza for the summer, and I couldn't wait for us to do this again.

Butterfly Effect

In 2011, I started working in a hospital. This was my third year after being diagnosed with Lupus. During this time, I was experiencing the butterfly rash across my nose, flare-ups on my arms, migraines, fatigue, and shortness of breath. When I was flaring up, it started to leave scars on my body and gradually changing my pigmentation. It wasn't anything I wasn't used to, but it was a lot to cope with. I had a rude awakening one day. Normally when I have migraines, they last for at least three days. But this day, I woke up with the worst feeling. I never experienced migraines like this before. This was a different feeling. Even though I felt this way, I still went to work. I was sweating, dizzy, and not myself. I was disoriented. As I was driving to work, I felt so hot, and I had the windows down, and the air conditioner was running simultaneously. I knew this was when I should have gone to the emergency room, but I had to get to work. I was thinking wrong, but I had a goal, and I did not want to miss any days.

I finally made it to work, and I could not concentrate on getting the report from the last shift. It was noticeable that something was going on with me. My director of nursing told me to rest my head for a while in the break room, and if I did not feel any better, to go to the emergency room downstairs. I was not going to go there because I was a private person. I did not want everyone to know what I had going on as far as my health. I did go to the break room to rest my head, but I did not get any better. Even my migraine medication was not working. It was this throbbing feeling behind my right eye that was just so heavy and unbearable. My director came to check on me and told me to go downstairs to the ER. I told her I would go down there, but I decided to leave and go home. This was another bad decision.

When I got home, I stripped immediately. I was so hot. I went and laid down. I thought that would help, but it didn't. I called my parents, who were at work. My father told me to call 911. I did call them, but I ended up right back at Northern Maryland Hospital. My parents did not live too far from there. They were about 7 minutes away. When I arrived at the hospital, I told them that I had Lupus, and they ran test after test and gave me a bag of fluids. After a while, the doctor arrived and told me it was just my Lupus flare-up. I needed to follow up with my Rheumatologist. I couldn't believe that was it. I asked myself if this was the part I needed to take seriously? This was a whole new ball game, and if this is it, I do not like this feeling, and I have children. I needed to start taking care of myself.

When I got back home, I went straight to bed. While I was asleep, I felt a throbbing feeling on the right side of my head. I could barely sleep, so I woke up and put an ice pack on my head, which would normally work. When I looked in the mirror, my right eye was slanted. It looked droopy, like I had a stroke. It was only on the right side. I went back to the hospital, but I went to County Hospital, where I received Lupus treatment. During this time, my children and I were living at my parents' house. I went to knock on my parent's room door to show them what was going on, and my father was the one who took me to the hospital.

Upon arrival, they rushed me in the back and took my vitals which were sky-high because I was in so much pain. They thought I had a stroke or was having a stroke. I was admitted right away. With County Hospital being a research hospital and my actual Rheumatologist being there, this is where I knew I would get the care that I needed. The testing alone was horrible. It was like I was going through delivery again because of the long needle they had to inject in my back to get fluid to see what was going on.

This was not a stroke because the right side of my body did not collapse or stop functioning. It was only the right side of my face. I was diagnosed with Tolosa Hunt Syndrome, a rare disorder that caused me to have a severe headache and unbearable pain in my right eye. This is caused by an auto immune disorder when you have Lupus. This caused my 5th nerve to collapse in my brain. That's why my right side collapsed. I became a guinea pig because this was rare, and only one case per million per year occurred in the United States. After five days, my eye and right side of my face became normal with treatment. I just knew that I was blessed, and I had to take my health more seriously than I was because if not, things could get worst. I was no longer just living for me but my children as well.

Juicy

There was another side of me that was hidden. A side that I never knew about until I met this man. In 2012 I was at the Exxon gas station, and when I was coming out of the store, there was this fine ass man. He was 5'11, and he was sexy. This man had caramel-colored skin, and umm my oh my, how I have a vivid vision of him as I tell this part of my life. I'm going to call him Juicy. He was staring me down with his eyes as if he was having sex with me. If I were him, I would want to have sex with me also. He didn't approach me with the normal, "Hey, can I get your number line" or "Aye Girl" line. He started with a joke and worked his way to him giving me his digits. Any other time another man could not get my phone number at a place where I lived across the street with Joshua. But I couldn't resist, it was friendly for now.

Joshua and I were not seeing eye to eye. If we, were I wouldn't be getting another man's number in the first place. If I were receiving the attention I needed at home, I wouldn't have placed myself in this predicament. Joshua was always with his cousins, especially his younger cousin. This grown-ass man was hanging with someone ten years younger than him every day. He was always gone and barely came home. We always argued about things he was doing around the house or what was not getting done. After being at work all day, I didn't want to come home to the unexpected. A breath of fresh air and something new wouldn't hurt.

It took me a week or so to call this fine-ass caramel man, but we started to hang out when I did. It was something about him, but I didn't know what it was. It felt special. Once I figured out what was so special about him, I loved it. He was passionate, loving, caring, loyal, and faithful. How can this man be all of what I was looking for? I couldn't give him anything in return because I was in a committed relationship, had a family, and the title and image of a committed relationship. He spoiled me and wanted to give me the world. I juggled two relationships with him and Joshua for a good two years. It was like the good and bad. We lived less than 5 minutes away from each other, so I would sneak out at night while Joshua was sleep. I treated him like a booty call. We hung out when we could, but it started to affect him. He wanted all of me and my time. I could not give him that. I didn't want to disappoint my parents because Joshua and I had been together for so long. We knew each other since we were 12 years old. But honestly, it was convenient and for an image. I was not in love with Joshua at this point. I only loved him. I gave him all that I could as a woman.

I worked hard, kept the house clean, had dinner on the table, and made sure the family was good. It was all left unrecognized, and I felt dismissed. This could have been the reason why I disrespected our relationship. Juicy gave me that other side I was looking for. He had flaws I could not deal with, like his unnecessary complaining and whining regarding our relationship because he wanted us to be together. One day my car broke down, and I had no other car to drive. Juicy decided to let me drive his car for the week while my car was down. I would leave out the house and walk across the street to meet him, drop him off at work, and run my errands or drop my kids off. I worked the night shift so that he would pick me up in the morning from work. This was a double life but something I could get away with. This showed Joshua paid no attention to the little details. Juicy and I was smooth sailing. I didn't have to worry about anything.

The second annual Luau party was also held this year. And this time, Eisha and I were both throwing it. But it was for Joshua's birthday. We had the party at Joshua's older sister's house. Everyone knew how the first Luau went, so I expected a big turnout. The bold side of me invited Juicy to the Luau. Yes, that's right! He was invited to the party that I was throwing for Joshua. I honestly did not think that he would come. I only invited him because he wanted to come so bad, asking me why I did not want him there? How weird is that? Juicy showed up but was very discreet on who he was. I acted as If he was just a guest whom I did not know; after all, this was an open invitation.

When we went on dates as far as going out to eat and movies, we had a meet-up spot. When it came to my health, he took care of me from a far but made me feel like I belonged to him. I did not want to end this. I wanted to leave and build my family with a man who I was falling for. This someone who loved me more than anything in this world, more than I loved him, but I had to snap back into reality. Time to cut the shenanigans. But how could I bring this to him, and how would this affect him? I wasn't sure, but I had to make it work between Joshua and me. I knew our love could be found or rebuilt because that was my best friend; we grew up together. He is the father of my children and took on responsibilities he did not have to take. I got into something with emotions, and now I was in too deep.

After breaking it off with Juicy, it was so hard. He was hurt. My thing was I had to make it work with Joshua and me for my family. Granted, this was a 10-year relationship of shacking up. In Maryland, we were married by common law. I gave Joshua a chance to see if things would change at home and had several conversations with him, but it was getting worst.

My cousin was graduating from Penn State. My kids and I were driving up state with my parents and siblings for this event. The night before, when I returned home, I had an unexpected guest. These were not my guest; they were Joshua's. This was one of the main issues I had with him; he did not respect his house. He acted like he lived on his own or had no family living with him. Anyways, it was his little cousin and his girlfriend, and their son along with the girlfriend's best friend. So as things were taking a turn, I decided to turn his ass out the door; I was livid. I called Joshua in the room to speak in private, and of course, he dismissed it. His excuse was he was tired, and it was late. I did not care how tired he was because he was leaving right out the door with all of them. The cousin's girlfriend's best friend had seen me a few days before coming to my house and never spoke to me; instead, she stared me down with mean mug looks. My woman's intuition signal came on. I always stayed one step ahead of Joshua. I always knew how he moved, but I could never prove it. The only way any of them was leaving was if Joshua would take them home, but he refused to due to him being so tired.

I allowed them to stay until morning because I knew I was going on this road trip up state with my family. Before I left early that morning, I woke everyone up, including Joshua, letting them know that their stay here was up and time to check out. Everyone left, and I cleared the house, so I thought. The trip was cut short because my father and directions in another state don't mix. The kids and I went straight home. When I got home, I heard voices in the back. I asked my kids to keep quiet. All I could hear was, "I can't find it," coming from my bedroom. When I went to the bedroom, it was Joshua and his cousin's girlfriend's best friend. That's right! My response to this lack of carelessness and stupidity act to the young lady was, "Did I not tell you to get the fuck out of my house?" She responded with, "What?" as she rolled her eyes and walked away from me. I blacked out and punched her in her face. Then I gave her an ass whipping right in my house, along with my son having her pinned up in the corner. I know I shouldn't have reacted that way in front of my kids, but this was a black-out moment, and my son did this on his own. Team works make the dream work at ten years old. I chased her ass out of my house as she screamed for help. She ran to Joshua's car where her best friend was waiting for her. I packed up Joshua's belongings because he had to go also.

Time went on, and I continued to see Juicy, but things were dying between us gradually. Joshua was staying at his sister's house, and I had to focus on grinding. There were times that I would be so stressed out, and I would flare up. This time around, it was not just affecting my skin, but it was the silent killer, which was my blood pressure, and it was uncontrollable. My mind was filled with so many emotions and playbacks that my body was starting to malfunction. I thought that I had elevated the issue but not enough to give me peace. Juicy thought we would be together because I asked Joshua to leave the house, but that was not my mindset. I may have wanted to build with him or love him, but my children came first. I could not put them in a place where they had to be around another man if they did not have to. The problem between Joshua and I could be fixed. There was no hatred between us. He's my kids' father, and I couldn't let this go for the sake of my children.

The time to end things with Juicy had come. I could only be friends and nothing more. I broke the news to him, but I had to carry on as if I didn't care. That's not how I felt. While I was ending things with Juicy, Joshua kept asking to come home. Either we both were going to make it work or walk away from it. Joshua decided he would come to the house to pick up some things, and when he came, he said we should get married. He didn't get down on one knee. Joshua had proposed to me in the past on one knee in the mall in front of the Kay Jewelers, and when we disagreed, well, big fight, I threw it. He replaced it with something bigger and better. We passed the mark of him proposing the traditional way. I said yes.

The announcement was being made that Joshua and I were going to get married. This was no surprise to the public but a surprise to me. Behind closed doors, things were not right between us. I mean, what women would not be excited to plan their dream wedding. Do not get me wrong; I was happy to finally focus on our relationship to fall in love again with my best friend. But shouldn't you be in love before getting married? When we spoke to my parents, they were happy, and for once, I felt like I did not disappoint them. I may not have given them a degree like my siblings did. But I had given them two grandchildren, and now my father can walk me down the aisle.

Pain

The date was finally set for September 13, 2014. I only had less than a year to get things going. In our relationship, there were red flags, but we were in a place that we both were content with. That was the problem. As a woman, of course, you have a load of planning, but you should still get the opinion of your future husband. That's what I thought. I don't know why I thought that because one of our biggest problems was, I always made the decisions.

One day while in bed, I had these weird pains in my lower back and stomach. These pains were indescribable and unbearable at the time. I asked Joshua to take me to the hospital, and we ended up arguing about who car he would take me in. I did not go to the hospital that night; instead, I bought meds that I thought would help with constipation because I thought I had to shit. That is exactly how I felt, torture and discomfort in my lower back and front of my lower stomach. I was sweating so hard like I have been in the sun all day. I laid on the bathroom floor crying in so much pain until one of the medications could work for me to pass a bowel. I hardly slept that night. I did not sleep at all.

The sun was rising, and birds were chirping. I knew I had no choice but to go to the hospital. Joshua had left for work, and the kids were gone as well. I crawled my way to the living room and broke down as if this was it for me. I ended up calling Eisha. I was crying so hard. I told her I felt like I was dying. She left work to come and get me. She must have passed all the lights getting to me because it felt like she got to me within 10 to 15 minutes. When Eisha arrived, she found me on my living room floor, balled up as if I were back in my mother's womb. She quickly helped me up and rushed me to the District Hospital.

Upon arrival, the wait was long. This hospital was always busy. When they finally called me to take my vitals, I went straight to the back. When the doctors checked me out, they found out that I had kidney stones and said I would have surgery if it did not pass through. Eisha stayed with me the entire time to make sure that things were getting done and contacting my parents. I was neutropenic, which means abnormal neutrophils in the blood, leading to increase infection, so sharing a room with another patient was out of the question. I stayed in the ER for three days. It felt like a week. The hospital had no beds available on the units. By the time they found me a bed, I was transferred and only stayed for two days. The stones ended up passing through without me needing surgery. For some reason, God was always on my side. I never doubted God, but I sometimes questioned things because of everything I had going on in my life.

Once I got back home from the hospital, I continued to plan my wedding. I felt like I was on the right track. I stopped seeing Juicy, and my focus was back on my family. Even with the minor hiccups with my health, things were getting done.

The Wedding

It was officially wedding time, and the planning was serious. I knew what my vision was and how I wanted everything to be. My maid of honor, bridesmaids, best man, groomsman, little bridesmaid, flower girls, page boys, usherettes, and godparents were chosen. I am the oldest of three, the first granddaughter to my grandmother on my mother's side, and the oldest granddaughter on my father's side in America. Well, that I know of. This was going to be an epic wedding. In our tradition, both sides of the family come up with the amount they will contribute as a family, meaning one household. For example, my father's side would contribute two hundred and fifty dollars each, but my mother's side of the family would contribute four hundred dollars, and that money would be put towards the wedding. I started to lose my pigmentation during the planning process, but it was not as noticeable, leaving a scar behind each time I flared up. The more I was thinking or was stressed, and my body would react to it.

My vision was brought to my childhood friend's mother, who was a decorator but made cakes as well. I trusted her, and I did not doubt in my mind she could make it happen. She introduced me to a wedding coordinator who I thought would be good to take the load off. Things were kind of hectic because you have two different cultures trying to put one wedding together. I was excited because I was able to choose and design my dress. Eisha and my sister were chosen for my Maid of Honors. Even though Eisha was my maid of honor, she was never fond of Joshua. This went way back to when we were kids. She knew we had that Martin and Gina love, so she went with the flow.

As a gift from Eisha, she paid for my dress. There was a budget set, and I had to work within that budget. Since I knew what I wanted, I made the budget work. From my dress to my vail and my shoes, it was everything I could imagine, and it was my vision. Everything was coming together, so I sat down with Joshua to get his input on things one day. I asked Joshua why he wasn't giving his input. It was OUR wedding. He had the nerve to tell me that I was forcing him. I immediately let him know if he didn't want to move forward to let me know, and I would shut everything down.

I called my mother, and she told me to take a step back. His family said he was getting cold feet. I never understood why a man would propose and then get cold feet. We finally cleared the air, and the wedding planning continued. The save the dates were being sent out, and my family planned a bridal shower. In our culture, a bridal shower is like a fundraiser. Everyone contributes money, and whatever the total is going towards your wedding. My family had t-shirts made with our pictures on them. Everything was just gorgeous. His side of the family was seeing how things were getting done. Yes, they have known me for the parties or doing things a certain way and knew that I was picky about how I did things, but now they are dealing with my family.

There was no participation from Joshua's mother's side of the family as far as the financial part or anything. But I did not expect that from them. I received participation from his father's side more than anything. They were the ones to deal with. The time was getting closer, and meetings were being called to finalize everything. I placed Joshua's sister in the wedding, but she was not cooperating. She didn't meet any deadlines, and she didn't show up to the meetings. I removed her from my bridal party, no questions asked. I have known his sister since she was six years old, and we never got along. We were cordial, and as time went on, we got older, we made it work, but, in her mind, I was not the one for her brother. She was disrespectful, and Joshua allowed that, but I was not going for that.

She always thought I was the problem in the relationship, not knowing that I was the responder. All I did was respond to Joshua's behavior. It may not have been the correct approach, but this was how I handled it at the time. The reason why she was placed in my wedding was for the sake of her brother. As time was getting closer and things were getting in place, I got nervous, not because I was scared but because I wanted things to be perfect. For the first time in a long time, I felt happy, and Joshua and I were back in a good space. Putting the time and investment in a relationship is a hell of a lot.

Our guest list was close to 500 people. My family was starting to arrive from all over the world. We had family from Australia, London, Atlanta, New York, New Jersey, Texas, and North Carolina. My family is big on both sides, so Joshua's family was beaten by three times. Everyone was excited, and I was stressed out because I was nervous. For my bachelorette party, the only thing I wanted to do was chill with my girls at the hotel, drink, and take my ass to bed. There was nothing or no one that was going to get in my way. We had come too far, and my mom sacrificed everything just for me to be able to do this. I was thankful for the parents God had blessed me with. My mother went above and beyond to make sure I had everything I needed. There was no room for error. I couldn't wait to see how everything came together. We had a U-Haul truck just to transport the food and liquor. The one thing that made me happy was bringing my father's side of the family together. They hadn't spoken to each other in over ten years, and my wedding brought them together.

It was time to say goodbye to Ms. Unpredictable. I was about to become a wife. The morning of my wedding came, and I was up and ready to go. The first thing I did that morning that I hadn't done in a while, thank God for life. That had to be my priority that morning. I was ecstatic because I made it to 28 years old. I was given multiple chances in life. This day was meant for me to walk down the aisle.

As I was getting myself together, there was a knock at my hotel door. My decorator had arrived with my bouquet in a beautiful fancy case. My wedding coordinator, make-up artist, and my girls were all ready to go. My princess felt like she should have been getting the same treatment as me. She wanted to feel like a little bride. While everyone was getting ready, I kept looking at the time. It seemed like there was no time left in the day. The time was moving so fast. We were all dressed, photos were taken, and the moment was finally here—time to meet my groom.

My palms were sweating, and my heart was beating as I stepped out of the limo to see my groom. He looked like he had seen a goddess walking through the doors. My soon-to-be husband was looking good. As I looked at him, I started to get butterflies in my stomach. I'll never forget that tingling feeling. That moment brought back memories of when Joshua and I first met. That was a great feeling to get back to. Everything was exactly how I pictured it. From the high ceilings to the king and queen chairs, centerpieces, and my cake. Absolutely breathtaking! The colors even made it look more like royalty with the gold and peach and all the African print in the orange family.

The music has started for the ceremony to begin. And for the first time, my father told me I looked beautiful. This had to be a dream, and I was surrounded by angels. I felt like a little girl all over again. As my father walked me down the aisle, I could see everyone whispering, smiling, sending messages, crying, and there goes Joshua in front of the altar with tears in his eyes. I would have never imagined him to shed tears of joy. I guess I couldn't expect everyone to be like me because I didn't cry tears of joy. We recited our vows, and now it was time to party with my husband. It was a long ceremony but worth it. Everyone was having a good time until my little cousin took the mic and announced that people's cars were getting broken into. The party was just getting started, but we celebrated until about three in the morning. We were showered with love and money all night. That was scratched off my bucket list.

Marriage

I was a married woman, and things were finally in place and done the proper way. At least at the beginning of our marriage. Why did I think that things were going to change because of papers or a title? In my eyes, it was only a contract. We had taken our vows in front of God and hundreds of witnesses. A few months had gone by, and my health started to take a toll on me. This is when you say, for better or worse comes, in-play. I started to go through the changes of hair loss, migraines, fingers turning purple from poor circulation called Raynaud's disease, and worst of them, all the red rashes that would turn into scabs and sores. A little cortisone or cream was not making it go away. It continued to mark my body gradually with discoloration. Fewer hours were getting put in at the hospital because I had been admitted to the hospital frequently.

The only thing I wanted to know was why my body was malfunctioning. I didn't know if it was all a mind thing or if my body was doing its own thing. I know I wasn't acting out of emotions; I didn't have a reason to. I didn't want to leave my job, or worst yet, get fired, so I decided to change shifts and units. I was going to stick with what I knew. Going to NICU/labor and delivery was a piece of cake, but some nurses were so fake. They were whispering on the low and chatting about my skin when I was going through the transformation. These educated but ignorant ass nurses had no clue. I mean, they thought I was contagious. They had the nerve to start questioning what I have. I started to have those feelings of insecurity. That was a feeling I had no idea about. I never had a reason to feel insecure until that period of my life.

I don't think people understood how I was feeling. I couldn't wear the clothes I like. I had to wear wigs because I was losing my hair. I always had to have a stock of makeup. I wonder if any of them would have wanted to switch places with me. Probably not! Therefore, they would never know how I felt. I never felt like I could not do my job, but these nurses made me not want to be around them. There were times I didn't even want to go to work. Despite my feelings, I refused to allow them to defeat me, stop me from doing my job, better yet, make me feel any kind of way because I was fighting for my life.

The decision was made by the doctors that I had to leave the health field officially. In December 2014, I had to walk away from what I knew. I didn't know what I was going to do. This was my world and all I had known since I was 19-years-old. I didn't know how I would be able to support my family. I knew I couldn't depend on my husband. We had not even been married for a year yet. He did what he could to provide, but as I said before, it was not enough. I knew he was not going to be able to handle this by himself. One thing I knew that I did not have to worry about was my children. He may have got on my nerves at times or had his childish ways, but he loved his kids.

When you love someone, they may not exactly be what you are looking for, and they come with flaws, but they will have good qualities about them. Joshua had good qualities. During our marriage, there was, but so much we both could take. When we had disagreements or arguments, things got out of hand most of the time. There was so much frustration and repetitive things occurring. He didn't have strong determination and was easily distracted. He always had a job and a car. But there were no leadership skills. No leadership skills, in my eyes, meant your character was weak. When I was forced to leave my job, Joshua's character was put to the test.

During this time, I was waiting for short and long-term disabilities. My mind was not at ease. I was restless and annoyed. Joshua started asking questions like what we are going to do about rent. He was waiting for me to handle everything. I was trying to figure out who had the balls in the marriage. I had too much on my plate.

I did receive my disability through work and hours from coworkers who donated their PTO to me. That pulled us through for about a year. Eventually, it would all have to come to an end, and bills were starting to pile up. We had rent, car insurance, buying household products, buying food out, and trying to maintain our social life. I applied for Social Security Disability which was a difficult process. I would hear things like they are going to deny me and that I needed a lawyer. I wasn't even worried because Eisha wrote a letter to the Senator of Maryland explaining that I was no different from other people experiencing the same thing. She wrote the letter to make them aware of another case in Maryland.

I was now experiencing the other side of depending on the government or, better yet, depending on someone to pull me out of the dirt. I was not used to this. My pride is too strong for a handout, but it had to be time. At that moment, I placed my pride to the side and thought about my family. At the time, we were living in Oxon Hill, and we were constantly late with the rent. I would go and speak with my rental specialist. Her name was Alysha. Anytime I would go into the office to speak with her, Alysha would make time for me. She was more than a rental specialist. Whenever I didn't have all of my rent, she would make sure we didn't get evicted. I remember one time when I was admitted to this hospital, and Alysha came to visit me. This was the type of person she was. It wasn't in her job description. She did it because she wanted to.

When I got older, I went to church but not as much as I was supposed to. The hardest part was getting up in the morning. In the back of my mind, there was a question always lingering. If God could constantly bless me, why couldn't I get up early one morning out of the week? I guess that is why I always wondered how I was always blessed.

After returning home from the hospital one time, things between Joshua and me were not good. We were back at stage one when the arguing and disagreeing would turn physical. Honestly, it was not Joshua being physical; it was me. I still couldn't control my anger. Sometimes Joshua would say stuff to hurt me. His words hurt me more than any physical touch. One time, he yelled out, "That's why he is not my son anyways." I was like, what. I never asked him to take on that role. He chose to do it. He requested for my son to call him daddy. That day I reminded him of that. Comments like that are what would cause the rage inside of me to come out. I couldn't have anyone, not even Joshua, say something like that out of his mouth. My prince was still unaware of who his biological father is.

You see, my Prince was incredibly special, both of my children were, but I gave him the protection that no one else in this world could give him but me. Whether I lived today or tomorrow, he was not wanted by the sperm donor and obviously would never be accepted. I allowed a man who was willing to step in as his father take the roll. If you want to hurt me, go ahead and say whatever you want to me but deny my son out loud for him to hear you were downright cold. I knew it was just him being spiteful to hurt me, but there are other ways to go about it. We were both fucked up to each other, but it was not in my character to hit below the belt with innocent children. My Prince was a blessing in disguise and how he entered this universe meant that he should be here. The only two people who can humble me and had the softest side of me were my children. They were my world. Everything I worked for was for them. I will always go above and beyond for them; they were not asked to be born. None of us were asked to be born.

It's Over

I kept my kids busy with activities. My son played football, and my daughter cheered. I dedicated time to them. Whether I was tired from work or even hanging out, I made sure I was there. My prince was good at what he did on the field. He had speed and always started. He played a running back position. His dedication to this sport was phenomenal. It was like he had a statement to make and took all his rage out on the field. On top of football, my prince still had his eye on being a firefighter. I still remember at the age of three, he knew he wanted to be a firefighter. As far as my princess, she had a big personality like her father. She loved to dance and show off. I used to play music while I was pregnant with her, and you can see her move around and kick. To me, she was dancing her way through the womb. She had the cheerleading thing down and was good at it. At six years old, she became captain of her squad.

My children are incredibly talented and highly intelligent. I never had an issue with schoolwork because they had that part under control. I played no games with their education. I took them to every practice and stayed out there with them. Joshua would make sure he showed up at their games. I did not want my kids to have idle time to hang around because that is how you get into the unnecessary stuff. I was not going to have them in the statistic group. Raising a young black man in America is not easy. With the help of my parents, my aunts, Eisha, siblings, and a few others, I do not know what I would have done during the downfall of my health and hard times.

Even though Joshua and I did not see eye to eye for better or worse right, I know I tried. He was staying out late and doing what he wanted to. His old habits never left. His ways caused me to revert to my old ways. We weren't even married for a year yet. We just crossed over to 2015, and things were rocky. He could say one word, and I would find a way to go off on him. I had no job, a disease in my body that was causing me to go through a physical change, raising my children and maintaining the household. This was all mentally challenging and just too much to bear.

I figured we should have passed this stage by now. We were married, and our marriage was being tested. I have shown my loyalty to this man I once was in love with. I fell out of love with him, and deep down inside, I made it work for the sake of my children. I know we should have gone to counseling or at least the pastor who married us. When we first went to marital counseling before getting married, she questioned whether we should get married or not. She saw the love there, but we were different and wanted different things. But with her advice and guidance, we made it through that stage. I may have messed around, in the beginning, going off my feelings of hurt or how things were not perfect at home, but once I said "I do," there was no turning back the hands of time until I started to suspect more than what I can handle. What Joshua had done to me and what I found out was unforgivable and put me in a place I could not walk away from. I started to walk away from everything that I vowed not to do as a married woman. Not knowing I would enter a world that would later in life put me in a place I always vowed not to be.

Malik was my cousin's best friend. I always thought he was cute. I thought he was dorky cute, but looks can be deceiving when you get to know him. My cousin was a male version of Eisha; we were close. We were a mirror image of each other. He was just black as tar, and I was caramel cinnamon. My cousin Sadique was dating Joshua's sister when they lived in the same complex as us directly across the street. Talk about the mirror in his relationship; he was going through his problems as well. If you left it up to Joshua and his sister, we planned this.

I called my cousin one night to see what he was doing. Sadique told me he was hanging out with his best friend, Malik and Brandon. They were about to ride their motorcycles. I was vulnerable at the time, so I said, "Oh, ask Malik when is he going to take me for a ride on his bike?" Malik was handsome, tatted, rode motorcycles, and dressed well. I was already attracted to him. Sadique then passes the phone to Malik for me to tell him myself. We exchanged numbers from there. By the way, he was in a relationship also. According to him, he was having issues and was trying to find a way out himself. It just sounds like a circle full of vulnerable people looking for that emptiness to be filled with love. At that time, it felt right because Joshua was not giving me the attention I needed at home.

One day Malik came to see me at my friend's house after I reached out to him. This was the first time we met up alone. Now I made sure I was on point in my jumpsuit. I was thicker than a snicker. My make-up was on point, and my all-white outfit. He was sweet, laid back, and I loved his swag. We started to see more of each other and hang out. We did what Joshua and I did not do, and that was date. It became late creep nights between Malik and me. It was an aura or a stench that he had that attracted me to him more. He would hit me up at night once he got to work, and he would ask me to come to see him. I would wait for Joshua to go to sleep. Once he was asleep, I got dressed and left out. I called myself the late-night creeper.

Even though Joshua and I were sleeping in the same bed, we were not having sex. I cut it off between us because I was just done with everything, and I would just be lying there if he asked me. Someone was showing me more than my husband was at the time. All kinds of thoughts were going through my head. Those questions were going through my head again.

Would God forgive me? Did he understand why I was doing this? I am his child. He can never deny me. He always had my back. What's the difference this time? I thought about all of that and still took my ass out the door once I received a message or a call.

When I would creep to see Malik, it would be around midnight because I would give him a grace period once he arrived at work at 11 pm to receive his report. He did security at an office building in the city. That was the only time we had to see each other because we both were in something. There were nights when we just hung out and sat outside of his job at the Starbucks table. Then there were nights when he would sneak me into the building, and I would go straight to the bathroom. We would have sex there and go about our night or go back outside and sit and talk. This reminded me so much of the sperm donor but in a different way. We weren't making love. It was just lust, and we had no ties to each other. We took our problems out in a sexual way. As time went on, we continued to pursue each other, and things started to get a little more serious. But we both knew it could not go but so far. Even with all the disarray between Joshua and me, I still had to play the wifey duty roles.

I was planning a small get-together pool party for his birthday. I always wanted to find a way to make things work with Joshua. My disability finally came through, which allowed some penny pinching so I could celebrate my husband's day. I was admitted to the hospital a few days before Joshua's pool party, so I canceled all plans. I guess everything happens for a reason.

During my hospital stay, Malik came to visit me. That was one of the things that stood out to me. Imagine being placed somewhere alone in a room, and throughout your stay, you are being poked and experimented on like a guinea pig. I would get admitted to the hospital frequently. Out of all the times I was there, which was like my second home, Joshua came at least twice but never slept in there with me. Joshua made time for what he wanted, and it wasn't me.

It was weird because Malik was one man with different parts of other men from my past. For example, he had a goofy side like Joshua, a sensitive side like Juicy, and a manipulative side like the donor. But overall, he showed me a side that he wanted more, and he wanted to build an empire and wanted to be wealthy like me. We also had things in common like motorcycles, cars, and tattoos. Those were my turn-ons.

When I was discharged from the hospital, I drove myself back home. That's how it happened sometimes. I would drive myself there and drive myself back home. When I got back home, I was not a happy woman. This was the day my mind was finally made up to walk away. I was having these feelings full of regret, but fighting temptations from my school love to my new love. I made up excuses for Joshua about not growing up in our relationship, and I was pulling the rope with him behind. He was a great person with a big goofy personality and smart but not great in our marriage. I don't even know why I got married. Oh yes, I do; it was for all of the wrong reasons. We had a family that involved children, he took the role of a father to my son when the donor never accepted him, and we went through everything together; he was my best friend. Instead of Gina and Martin, we became Ike and Tina, with me being Ike.

At this time, I had so much built-up anger, animosity, and frustration to unleash. I was already hurt from a situation I could never forgive him for, and I could not get that out of my mind. That vulnerability is what led me to Malik in the first place. It may sound like excuses, but I was a woman who was scorn. I made it clear to Joshua that I was putting in a 30-day notice, and at this time, I could care less who had something to say. I was tired of babysitting or sounding like a broken record. I guess he took me for a joke, but I walked my ass across that street the next day and handed over my notice to Alysha. I let her know I appreciated her for everything she had done for my family and me, but I would no longer be residing there. I explained to my children we were going to stay with my parents for a little while. Telling my kids we were leaving hurt me. I put a lot of work into our time together. But I left with no remorse. Malik had my attention now.

Joshua thought I was joking because when those 30 days had come, he didn't pack anything. I was packing since the day I told him I was leaving. When it was time for us to move, Malik was there to help. Joshua had no idea what was going on between us, but he didn't come alone. My cousin and their other best friend were there to help me move my things to storage and my parents' house.

Before moving back home, I had to speak to my parents about what was going on. My parents had no idea what was happening in my marriage. The situation was out of control, and I needed them. My father told me I could come home. He assured me this was always my house. He supported me 100%, but my mother was a different story. She was not happy. My mother told me I couldn't come home because I needed to make my marriage work. I couldn't blame her because she was right. It wasn't even a whole year, and I was walking away. I had brought shame to my family. That's the only reason I stayed for as long as I did. But I was tired, and I no longer cared. I was her daughter, so she didn't have a choice. My parents never turned their back on me. I knew the disappointment was there, but she wasn't going to turn me away. I would explain everything to her later.

Once I arrived back home to my parents, I had some explaining to do. Not really to my father because he backed me up. It was like he wanted me home anyways. My mother was so disappointed with me. The look on her face was as if I destroyed her entire world. It hurt me to the core, but I needed her to understand that I could no longer be there. That environment was not good for my children. I did not want them to continue hearing the arguing and the fighting. I kept getting sick with flare-ups, and my blood pressure was a major problem. I did not know how to control myself and before either one of us did something we would regret, I would rather walk away. She still didn't understand and was upset with me. Mad or not, I stuck to what I said and didn't budge.

My mother wanted us to have a sit down with Joshua and his mother. I agreed to sit down, but I didn't care, and I wasn't going back. We had the meeting, and nothing worked. The thing about Joshua was that he lied, not thinking someone would find out the truth. He claimed he was sleeping in the car when we left. He had already moved in with another woman. Those times when his ass was not coming home, he was already doing his dirt. This was before I even decided to step out in our marriage. In my eyes, we were even. There was no turning back, and I patiently waited for a year to file for a divorce. It would have taken a miracle for our marriage to work. This had nothing to do with Malik. I felt how I felt.

Blended

As time went on, I broke my code. I was big on not bringing multiple men around my children. I don't know what I was thinking this time. Malik had a son. At the time, this was his only child. I had not officially met him when I would go to Malik's mother's house, but I would see him walk past and peek here and there. My Prince was playing football when both he and my daughter had just started on another team. I told Malik that they had tryouts because he had told me that his son wanted to play football. I didn't think he would bring him, but he fooled me.

It's 2016, and Malik and I have now gone from just kicking it to a monogamous relationship. I still wasn't divorced, but my year was almost up from my separation. My apartment was ready for me to move in. At the time, Malik was living with his mother, so when it was time for me to move in, he and his son came along. Everything was moving so fast. I couldn't believe it myself. Things I wouldn't normally do, I was doing it. I was always the head of the household or the one who would decide the relationship, but I didn't have to for the first time. I didn't have to figure everything out this time around.

Once he moved in, I was too far gone. My body was filled with butterflies, and I was floating on cloud 9. I was determined to make this work. I was truly in love. Living with him felt like I had just met him for the first time. I was thinking to myself one day about how I must have lost my mind, letting him move in. I laugh now because I am an alpha female. I am the leader of my wolf pack. But I didn't have to be that way with Malik.

Eisha knew something was up. She was starting to see a change in me that she had never seen before. From the first time she even knew we were dating, she said to me, "It's something about him. He is sneaky, and I don't like it. Are you sure you know what you are doing?" Maybe I should have listened to her then. But these signs that were being told to me were overlooked. By Malik and Sadique being best friends, he went with the flow. He didn't get in the mix because he had his relationship with Joshua. They were not best friends, but they respected one another. Joshua just felt like Sadique put Malik and me together when he had nothing to do with it.

Our kids started playing on the same team. Our boys played football with their age group, which was 6u and 14u. And my daughter was a cheerleader. Our children seemed to get along, and we were at all the games together along with Eisha, Sadique, and his mother, who called my children her grandchildren as well. When she and I first met, she told me that she let Malik know she did not want to meet me unless we were serious. At least, that is what she was hoping for or told me.

The way our kids met was weird. Malik decided to bring his dog to the park one day, and he was not a small dog neither. He was a pit. His dog attacked a smaller dog, and I thought his ass was going to swallow him for lunch. He got a whiff of that sucker and was on attack mode. I had them place the dog in my car and drove off from the park so Malik would not get into trouble or have his dog taken away. He grabbed all of the kids and met his cousin and me at the gas station to get the dog from me. I am not sure how he felt after, but I know it was nothing for me to have his back. That was in my blood.

We lived together for a few months, and things became crazy when we disagreed. Malik would ignore me and not speak. That got under my skin. I don't like the silent treatment. I felt like every step was a part of a puzzle in shambles, and I was trying to put the pieces back together. One day we had a falling out about something that I thought was blown out of proportion. He didn't speak to me for a day or two. I went to work one day, and I was looking forward to going home. I thought it was time to break the ice. Little did I know what I was walking into once I got home. I opened my front door, and my apartment was empty. The only thing left in there was my big screen television, my mattress, and the kid's beds. I immediately shut the door to see if I was in the right apartment. It was my door number. I know I didn't get robbed. I found out this man had moved everything out. Granted, it was his living room, dining room, and bedroom furniture, but this showed me to have my own. That situation didn't make me feel good as a person. The only thing I had left was my television on a stand and my kids' bed. This fool took everything back to his mother's house. All because of a disagreement. More red flags that I continued to ignore.

I got in my car and was driving in rage. I was boiling so much inside that I could feel the heat in my body. I was talking to myself and everything. What did I get myself into, and how would I react when I saw him? When I arrived at his mother's house, my children and his son sat outside talking to their grandma. By this time, my kids called her grandma, and his son called me ma. This was all a twisted soap opera. Finally, regrets started to sink in so deeply that I just broke down in tears. Malik's mother and I had a relationship outside of ours. I was closer to her than I was with my mother-in-law. She made me feel so comfortable and gave me hope. She was sweet, kind, and always prayed for us. She accepted my children and me as her own.

When I arrived, she asked me to come in so that we could speak. She wanted to get my side of the story. She explained that we had to let each other cool down and things will work out. The kids had a football game the next day, but I could not sleep, eat, or think. I just knew I was going to have a flare-up and was going to be sick. I was right. I tried everything so I wouldn't have to go to the hospital. I didn't want to miss my kid's game. Eventually, I still ended up in the hospital, which Malik was the one who took me. We spoke about it, and he did return the furniture to the house. There was no reason why I shouldn't have had my furniture in that apartment. I let my guard down for the first time.

When Joshua and I separated, I placed our furniture in storage, but I end up letting everything go. I wanted a fresh start, so Malik had furniture at his mother's house and guaranteed me that there was nothing to worry about on that end. I had no reason why I shouldn't have trusted him. I did learn my lesson from this as time went on. I started to become more observant with him.

Envy

My children had been used to a stable household and always lived with Joshua and me under one roof as a family. I may have done my dirt in the past, but I worked hard to provide for them. But I couldn't do everything by myself. Joshua did the best he could as a father, no he was not perfect, but he loved our children, and I knew he loved me. I wanted him to feel the hurt I felt. I wanted him to see that I didn't care. I had to face the truth. It was what it was.

He would still get the kids when he needed to. But I made it clear when it came to my kids and his girlfriend. I do not care what part of you she may have, but one mistake with my children, and her world is over. He never approved of Malik being around our children, neither. But our children liked his girlfriend, and I never heard neither one say anything negative about her. My only concern was to make sure my children were happy because they were experiencing a split home and new faces.

I received a phone call one day from Joshua telling me he needed to speak with me. We may have had our crazy side, but we had always been friends first. He had always been comfortable talking to me when he needed advice, even when we were younger. When we spoke on the phone, he sounded nervous, and his voice was a little shaky, but he finally came out and told me that he was expecting a baby with his new girlfriend. I was not expecting this news. I was quiet for a bit, but I asked what they were going to do. He said to me that he did not want to have another child. And that he already told her how he felt. I told him it was her choice because she was carrying the baby.

I wanted to have another child once we were married, but Joshua told me that he did not want another. My health was already screwed, but I figured we could have one last one. I had been pregnant six times in total, including my two children. I had two abortions and two miscarriages. I could not hold my pregnancies due to me being diagnosed with lupus. The medication I was on was an immunosuppressant pill, and I received it by IV. If I were to get pregnant, chances are the baby would come out deformed. Joshua sounded scared and confused, but it was easy for me to let him know he had my support because he felt very strongly about not keeping this baby. But his girlfriend also felt otherwise. So, they kept the baby. At first, I didn't care, but it started to anger me in ways I did not expect, especially when I would see her. But my focus was now shifted to building my own family. Maybe a miracle would happen. When something is meant to be, God will make a way.

Division

My relationship with Eisha became complicated because she was dating Joshua's first cousin, Phil. Eisha owned a condo, a nice car, and had a good job. When Phil got with Eisha, he became big-headed. He had a job doing security, but big things started for him when he was dating Eisha. He began traveling, he had a nice car, a dog, and he enjoyed life. But when the arguing started or disagreement between the two occurred, it was like Tyson and Holyfield. They did not work out, and Eisha broke up with him. Our relationship became complicated because when they broke up, I continued to be friends with Phil. After all, we had our own friendship. When Joshua and I had our first place together, Phil stayed with us for a while and helped take care of our kids. He helped raise our daughter that was his rent. Eisha didn't like that I remained friends with Phil. Even though she wasn't happy, we are in a better place now.

To be in a world of love, you must be prepared to enter through the gates of heaven or hell. Love is a treacherous word to use when you are in an intense, deep romantic or erotic attachment. It is like your mind, and the intensity in your body has no control. While you are in heaven, there are positive psychological effects on your daily life. At the beginning of a relationship, there's lust for the first year. Then, it's the intensity of sex, pillow talk, and being around each other. That was how I felt about Malik in the beginning. I was head over heels when we were dating. Entering hell was the second year of our relationship when both character's true identities begin to show. The disagreements, accusations, and sneakiness begin to unravel. The insane part was that I was 100% faithful to this man. No one could get my attention or even my time. The time, energy, and compassion that I gave in the relationship should have said it all. When you are not doing the creeping, you become the suspect, getting falsely accused. I was starting to feel like this was a liability. But I wasn't going to give up. All eyes were on my parents, family, and friends. The biggest thing would have been the disappointment of my children. That would destroy my world more than anything.

Bringing our children under one roof was not an easy task. It was rocky. When I first met Malik's son, I wanted to build my relationship with him, but I wanted it to come gradually and naturally. We both had a genuine love for each other because he began to call me Ma on his own. I was astounded. It made me feel great that he would give me that title. His mother was still in the picture, and I never wanted to step in her position. I was just a bonus.

When our children met, things were good, but there were plenty of disagreements and pointing fingers as time went on, which started to affect Malik and my relationship. My daughter loved Malik; my daughter started to call him Dad. From there, I knew that this would be an issue once it got back to her father. This was a new world for my kids. They had already been through enough with the separation and divorce. Now adding an addition to the family and getting adjusted would be a job of its own. So I dug into my children's world by changing their routines. I mean, I changed their schools to where Malik's mother lived so that she was able to help both of us while we worked. I was just all in his world, but I thought we were both on the same page. My daughter attended his son's school, and my son attended school in that area as well. Of course, they weren't happy about that, but this was an adjustment for all of us.

Now that the children are all somewhat adjusted to their new school and home, things were going better than expected. This was just temporary. Eventually, Malik and I were not seeing eye to eye when it came down to certain things with the kids. Malik was the type to throw things under the rug instead of discussing them. And I was the type to hold things in. When it was time to discuss it, I would explode, or it would come out wrong.

My Prince was older at the time. He was about 15 years old. I never had a discussion with him about Joshua not being his biological father. But when Malik and I got together, I expressed to him how I felt about that. You see, in my eyes, I was protecting my son from the truth because I did not want him to get hurt, knowing that the sperm donor had made it clear to me that he did not want to be a part of his life. But it was not about me. It was about my son. When I was still in high school, I believe I was in the 10th or 11th grade, only one person reached out to me, and that was the sperm donor's first daughter, mother. She also attended District Heights high school but had graduated from there already.

One day she came to the school and picked me up and took me to her place. We sat and talked as women. She never once pushed me away, made me feel uncomfortable, or treated me like a little girl. I explained to her how I felt and what my situation was. She told me when I was ready, she was willing for her daughter and my son to meet as siblings. I always thought about it but was too afraid to do so because I never told my son the truth. With Joshua and I no longer together and with Malik in the picture, the truth would eventually come out. Finally, Malik convinced me to talk to him. This was not the first time I was told to have this conversation with my son. Eisha told me to have this conversation with him because it would hurt him more if it didn't come from me.

As I was planning to tell my son the truth, I guess he beat me to the punch. One day we were out, and we found a letter with him expressing how he felt. He knew the truth all along. In his letter, he expressed how his cousin on Joshua's side

93

had told him that Joshua was not his father. My son was around six or seven at the time. He also said he would hear Joshua and I argue, and comments would be made from Joshua saying, "That's not my son," or "he's not my son anyways." Joshua said those things when he was upset with me. The thoughts and emotions running through my blood, brain, and head were scattered and embarrassing. Malik and I were a team, but this is my child, and there were things in the beginning that Malik didn't need to know. I didn't think this was his issue.

My concern was my son, and I knew I needed to fix this. The last thing I needed was everyone's opinion. In all honesty, I did not know how to respond, but I had to have a one on one with my child. I had to tell him how much I loved him, and I didn't mean to hold this secret. It wasn't my intention to hurt him. I only wanted to protect him. As a mother, I felt like I had everything under control and that by me prolonging or procrastinating to tell my son the truth about his father, he would understand. I was clueless because kids know everything, and they sometimes hold it in. I just hoped and prayed my son would forgive me and understand why I did it.

Malik did step in and talk to him about the situation. Eventually, he did build a relationship with my son, but that didn't last long. When you make promises to children that you can't keep, it's a hurtful feeling. But, there's a difference when you don't have control over the situation versus when you intentionally hurt a child.

Sometimes things happen, and we have so many doubts and crazy thoughts in our heads on how it should have played out or what could have happened. In this situation, it was a process, but eventually, we worked through it, and I had to rebuild the trust between my son and me again. But what I did not know was that this would be a long road not for my son and me but overall, just trying to have a blended family.

I know what I said about me not caring about what people had to say, but deep inside, I still cared.

My cousin Eisha had gotten married in 2016, and my daughter and I were in her wedding. In my eyes, we were still that duo that was unstoppable, but this was when loyalty, respect, and trust all factored in. I was one of her Maid of Honor's along with her best friend. I was honored to be at her wedding. I wish that she would have gotten married when I could do more or at least work. As one of her Maid of Honor's, my job was to be her right hand, but sometimes that right hand felt handicapped. I love her. I should have been able to do double of what she did for me when I had gotten married. But the timing was bad. I was not bringing in much because I was receiving disability and picked up a front desk job at an agency. My flare-ups were getting worst. I had gained so much weight in my face. It was fluid because I was placed on Prednisone steroids. My weight and emotions were all over the place. Her wedding time was approaching, and things were starting to unravel. After all, she is more than a cousin. She is my sister.

Malik and I were on shaky ground, and he officially moved out. Malik was making excuses such as there were bad spirits in my apartment. He would lie and say that when we got into an argument, I asked for my keys back. That was all bullshit. That was only an excuse for him to go back to his mother's house. He wanted to have his cake and eat it too. That should have been my exit to leave, but of course, I was stuck on making it work between us because I had already given up on my marriage. That didn't mean I had to keep taking his accusations and womanizing behavior. He took the coward way out and found a way for me to blow up on him and finally leave.

We were at a track meet, and he was acting funny like he did not want to be around me. He was acting as if he was so busy on his phone. This man stayed in his car and was just talking on the phone while I was at his son's track meet. After the track meet, I decided to approach him. We both got loud, and I said I did not want to be with him. In the heat of the moment, you say things you do not mean, but I believe I felt that way but did not want it to come out like that. Fuck it! It was out, and there was no turning back the hands of time. We were already in our separate spaces. It was just time to let it go.

We broke up. In my eyes, he was looking for a way out. He should have been honest about how he felt. I felt like I was placed in a position that I could not get myself out of. But if I could get over my marriage without looking back, then I can do the same here. I didn't know if it would be that easy because I was in love. Love hurts. I made my bed, so I needed to lay in it. Even though it was right in front of my face, I still was foolish.

Four months had passed, and I had started gradually moving on. My children and I had moved and settled into our new home. It was 2018, and I had just lost my grandmother. Even though I only met her once, I always felt so close to her. Out of the three of us, I am the child without a middle name. Since I didn't have a middle name, I renamed myself using her name as my middle name.

Malik reached out to me because he heard about my grandma's passing. When I saw the number calling, honestly, I was not going to answer. It was only because I spoke to his mother when she gave her condolences. She asked me if it was okay for Malik to call me, and I said yes. I had blocked that ass. That is how I moved on. I unblocked him to receive the call, and he sent his condolences to my family and me. I knew once I heard his voice, I would reverse, but I had to be strong. Not just because I was upset or hurt, but my children were hurt by the breakup as well. I failed because I didn't see how the children felt about our breakup. We should have talked to them about it. After Joshua and I divorced, Malik was the other man in their life. It was broken promises after broken promises. My son found out Joshua wasn't his biological father, I talked to him about the sperm donor, and Malik failed promises; made me feel bad as a mother.

After speaking to him, the texting started back up again. Slowly but surely, we were back at it again. After we broke up, he was in another relationship. That's why he kept making up excuses as to why he needed to leave. Even though I knew that I was contradicting myself. I was right back there where I shouldn't have been. Men move on quickly without looking back, while women are still trying to mend a broken heart. While he was in this relationship, he had gotten her pregnant. I was given the option to either stay and work it out or let it go. Of course, I was the damn fool that stayed. I was loyal to him. I brought him back around my children and family. He was making a mockery out of me, but I couldn't walk away. I did the bid with him the entire nine months of her pregnancy. I lived in my place, and he had his. I might have been a fool for him, but I wasn't that stupid. I was barely at my place. I was like a dog marking her territory.

Malik told me they were not messing around. They strictly communicated because of the baby. I didn't buy it. He was moving like a fox. That was his spirit animal. She would call numerous times a day, and when he went to the appointments with her, his ass was ghost. He always thought I did not know what was going on, but I was fully aware. A woman would not call you numerous times asking you where you are or who you are with, getting mad when you do not answer the phone, and always need you for the littlest things if something wasn't going on. But I couldn't complain because that was all on me. I took him back. I thought if I stuck it out and supported him, he would recognize it. It got so bad he would put her needs before mine, which made me more aware that something was still going on.

I am a true believer in karma. I would know because of all of the shit I had done. When his new baby arrived, it was hectic for a while, not that bad but bad enough. I couldn't believe I stuck it out with him for nine months. The baby did not ask to be here. She was innocent. I helped take care of her as I should because we were together. But everything was a secret to the mother. She and I never physically met, but we knew about each other.

When he finally told her that we were together, all hell broke loose. She would barely allow him to get his daughter. And the times he did get her, he acted like he was still living at his mother's house or watching her over there. He was bringing her home the whole time, or he would watch her at his mother's house. I would help watch or take care of her 80% of the time. When there were disagreements between the two of them or they were not getting along, I was the one sending the text messages and communicating with her as though I was him. I was acting like I was in the market to buy love. The things I was doing. He would always lie to her and tell her one thing, which caused many mix-ups. Mix-ups always occurred. He would lie to her and tell her one thing and do the same with me.

We decided to move back in together, but I was skeptical and certain it would work out simultaneously. I know it sounds crazy, but what we have been through and sacrifices made on both ends made it look like it would work. Everyone was excited to see our little family together again.

Caught Up

After two weeks of moving in together, our happy home became a broken home. Malik was moving sneakily again, but this time I would compare him to a lion. No need to worry because so was I. One day he said he was going out and would be back. I knew he wasn't going to hang out with his boys. I already got a whiff of his bullshit. It is a small world, and people are always watching even when you think they are not.

Malik slipped up a few times, not knowing I was soaking in all the crap he gave me. He always brought up this one female named Nicole. Every time he brought Nicole's name up, I counted. Nicole was his supervisor. Before we moved back in together, he was caught texting and talking to her late at night. I mean, there is nothing professional about how they are communicating. When he was caught, he admitted he was flirting and communicating with her, but nothing happened. When Malik was going through something major in his life, I stuck by his side through it all. None of these women were there when he was going through a rough patch.

One particular night he was going out supposedly with his boys. I waited for at least two minutes and googled her first and last name. I got her address, and I was out the door. I was on my Carmen San Diego bullshit. I needed to see for my own eyes that I was not losing my mind. Before leaving out the house, I took a gun from out of the safe. I was not thinking, but this was all off emotions. I didn't have far to go either because she lived around the corner, less than six minutes away from us. As I got closer, I begin to talk to myself. I was hoping I wouldn't see his car or catch them together. As I pulled into her complex, the first car I saw was his. There's an old saying if you go looking, you find. I found him at another woman's house between the hours 11 and 12 midnight. I knew there was nothing professional about that.

I immediately started to go off. I was asking God why did he lead me here. I blacked out and went code red. I kindly parked and waited to cool off. I also waited to see if I was going to catch him coming out. There was no sign of him, but his car was there. To get into the building, you needed a code. At first, I wasn't able to get into the building, but my miracle showed up. Someone was there right on time to open the door. I lied and told the man I was locked out of my cousin's house. It was all lies, and the devil was working overtime that night. Even with the stuff I went through with Joshua and the donor; I never felt this angry. I saw sparkles and red. I was in too deep. I continued walking through her building with my gun, and I knocked on her door. No one would answer, so I continued to bang. All I could hear was a dog barking. At some point, I thought I heard footsteps. I don't know what I heard, but my mind was gone.

Even with the devil working that night, God worked harder because he sent two people my way to calm me down. Between his mother and my cousin talking to me on the phone, I don't know what would have happened. They both convinced me to turn around. When I returned to my vehicle, all I could do was break down and cry once the adrenaline high came down. The feeling of hurt and disappointment but the expectation at the same time was something I never experienced.

I reached out to the supervisor he was sneaking around with. I found out we knew each other. We talked, and supposedly she did not know about me, but I didn't believe that. I gave her the benefit of the doubt. That was all I gave her. They continued to see each other, and by this time, Malik had one foot in and one foot out. I have never seen a man in a relationship, living at home with his girlfriend and kids, with them seven days a week, and still creeping. Five out of those seven days, he told me he was at his mother's house.

I should have expected the worst to come my way. I spoke to this young lady at least twice that I can remember vividly. The second time I spoke to her, I called her again within two months of Malik being caught. This time I pulled phone records to see for myself. Love will have you do things you just could never imagine yourself doing. I drove to the Tmobile store and saw a young girl working there that I thought could use some extra money for lunch. I pulled her to the side and told her I wanted to pull phone records on my cheating boyfriend. I proceeded to tell her I will pay her $40 to pull the records. She hesitated a while, but she did it. I wasn't surprised at anything I found as far as the late texting and phone numbers. This was bound to happen and was a form of karma. Unfortunately, the grass was not greener on the other side. It was brown as hell.

After pulling the records, I called her again, asking if she was still dealing with him, and she told me she was. I was done competing with her. He was hers to keep. This is deeper than I even thought. He was telling both of us things, and I believed everything he was saying. I allowed too much to go on and left many things unsaid because I wanted to make it work so bad. I knew my worth, but I didn't value it. I called Joshua weak, but I was the weak one in this situation all because of an image. I didn't want to look like a failure to my family.

Stress is the number one factor that will trigger my flare-ups. Around this time, I was getting extremely sick. I was in and out of the hospital with my blood pressure increasing. This time when I was discharged, I could tell he was acting differently. He was very nonchalant. I kept asking him what was going on, and his response was nothing, but the lion was preying on his food. I continued to ask until I received an answer. With a roll of his tongue, he told me he was expecting a baby with this girl. My heart came out of my ass. He just didn't care about me at all. How I felt didn't exist. There was no name for it. The audacity of this man to sit on my bed and come out of his mouth after being home a few hours and tell me something like that. I asked him to tell me, so he gave it to me. If deceiving were a person, he would be it.

This man not only got one female pregnant while we were together, but there was also a total of three. He shared himself with the world. You would never know he was a womanizer. He just fed everyone lies. He was a lion preying on his food, and he ate my ass up.

Scandal

Malik and I never worked out but were still having sex. We had broken up, but I continued to sleep with him. At that point, I could care less about how someone felt because no one thought about me. I despised him and didn't trust him or anyone else. I wanted him to feel what I felt, so whatever was his consequences I could care less. He took my character and made me look like a fool. I never once cheated on him. The saying "how you got him is how you will lose him" that was me. Overall, he was with who made him happy. A man knows what he wants within six months of meeting someone. I gave him four years that I will never get back. Time wasted. He had several times where he could have exited out the door. In the end, he was caught by his supervisor friend that we were still sleeping with each other. He solved that problem by proposing to her with the ring he supposedly had for me. He was a reflection of me. He taught me that karma is a bitch. All that I have done in my past with Joshua because I was responding to his acts with Juicy or just holding on to imaginary love was brought back to me.

This was the first time I experienced depression. I was depressed and battling a disease. I wouldn't wish this on my worst enemy, even if it was Malik and the sperm donor. The feeling of loneliness, emptiness, and defeat was worse than the war I was in. I did not eat, barely slept, and was so hidden I started to lose myself. I was ashamed to face my family. I was not hanging with anyone because I built everything around my little family. My vexation came from how Malik went about it. I would have respected him more if he was honest about how he felt.

If someone is not happy, do not continue to lead them on and give false hope of a future. My hurt came from allowing this man to manipulate my mind with these promises that he could not keep. As he displayed these acts, I ignored them and went with the words he whispered in my ears. It all sounded like music but coming from a broken record. I thought about doing what I did when I was pregnant by the sperm donor. I wanted to overdose on medication. I thought about it, but I didn't. I was tired of going through so much. Then he had the nerve to drag my name in the dirt as if he walked away as the victim. That was amusing to me.

At the end of 2019, all the hell and fire I had been through finally passed me. It took some time, but I haven't been through anything in my life that I couldn't defeat. I learned a very valuable lesson, and that is to love myself. It was in my head that I was not who I was before. I have grown to be a woman who needed to learn self-love and needed to learn how to walk away. I couldn't continue being a be a people pleaser. Red flags are signals of what you should pay attention to and the words they use. Action speaks louder than words. Many times, those actions are false advertisements.

The Rise of the Phoenix

I always felt like I was changing gradually as I continued to fight through this battle with Lupus. My body was really at war with bombs located in different sections of my body, from the top layer of my head to my chest, hands, back, and hips. My flare-ups were leaving scars of pain that Cocoa Butter could not remove. My flare-ups were so bad that I had to be admitted to the burn unit. My hands were changing to pink due to the pigmentation; my back was four different shades; I lost my hair and became someone I could not recognize. This made me feel very unconfident. I couldn't even recognize myself when I looked in the mirror. I broke down from tears of sorrow inside and out. I kept asking God how long would I be in this war of torment. I was always the showoff, and I loved to show skin. Now all I want to do is cover myself. I believe in my heart that was one of the main issues in my relationships. Not everyone can handle it, and it was just too much to deal with. It was never about past relationships; it was about me—I lost myself.

I thought 2020 would be the year of vision, but it came with more than an open eye. I was back working, but this time as an Insurance Agent. This job required you to meet the client at their homes and go door to door knocking. I was unable to do the job after being there for three months. Then, I started to notice excruciating pain in my hip. One day I was going into the office, and I could not walk. It was a struggle. I ended up showing up to work with a cane. That feeling was not good. There were no feelings at this point. My body had become numb to things that were occurring to me.

I went to the doctor to get an x-ray to see what the problem was. When the doctors were back with the results, they told me that I would need surgery, and I had Avascular Narcosis, which is associated with long-term use of steroids and drinking too much alcohol. In my case, it was the steroid use which I have been on Prednisone for over 11 years, and it affected my hip. I was no longer surprised when it came to anything with my body. Bad news should be music to my ears. This was a whole new journey to be in, and at this point, it did not matter who, when, or how it was coming. I started my new year with surgery which was in January. It was for a right hip core decompression. This surgery was done to bear the pain, meaning buy me time not to have a hip replacement at 33 years of age. Both sides were done within a two-month span which is an in and out surgery.

Three months after the surgery, I had to get my left hip replaced. Before the replacement, I still felt that excruciating pain on both sides. The doctors had always explained to me that the surgery could or could not work. So, in June, I did the same surgery on the worst side, which was the right side which gave my doctor another chance to fix things. I trusted him and his work because he gave me the full details of what the surgery would come with. It worked for some time on the right side. Then the left had to be replaced. The fourth surgery was done in August to replace the left hip.

I was in so much agony after surgery. I was not able to get in and out of bed. I couldn't even walk up and down the steps. I depended on others like my sister and mother to take care of me for two weeks and Sadique's finance. From cooking to cleaning, they made sure I was in good care. The healing process was supposed to be 10-12 weeks. My turnaround time was in six weeks. I was motivated and determined not to be using this handicapped equipment. I woke up every day at the same time to take a shower, get dressed, and go down the steps as if I was going to work, but I was doing therapy and writing. My goal was to get back on my feet before the time given and come back even stronger. That goal was met, and I got back on my feet even stronger than before. However, all good news must come to an end. My right-side pain arrived again. Now I had to replace my right side so that both hips could be even and at ease.

There was a time in my life it was so easy to get dressed. There was no hesitation or having difficulties finding what to wear. In the past, there was not much to cover. As I said earlier, I love to show off, and that's skin too. But it has not been easy to be comfortable in my skin since the scars on my body had started spreading like wildfire, along with the physical change. This pushed me deeper into a hole where I never wanted to come out of. So many mixed emotions from happy, sad, sensitive, and angry. One thing about me I would never show true feelings. I could not show the world my weakness. But all I was doing was hurting myself, continuing to bottle up all my feelings. I became insecure, always having to cover my arms. I couldn't even wear short sleeves to go to the gas station or go outside to check the mail.

This experience has been strenuous. Having one of your senses taken away from you was something I just could not envision. My world was something dissimilar to the world I was born into. Step into my shoes for a day. Imagine going to sleep, and deep down, you're wondering if you will wake up the next morning to see your children. Or imagine having people constantly asking you what happened to your skin, whether you were burned by fire or have vitiligo, or even just staring at you. The worst is crying every day and watching your kids grow because you don't know if you'll see them become parents. I went from having surgery to barely walking, walking with a cane, bedridden, to being back on my feet. It's not easy, but I'm strong.

From everything I have been through in life, the people I have encountered, and the negative and positive experiences I had, I thank every person for playing their role. Without having those experiences, I would not be the person I am today. I transformed from the Phoenix risen from death. I had so many battles that most people wouldn't survive. I gave birth to my son when I was 15, and I almost died. My son is now 18 years old and currently preparing for the fire department. I was married and divorced shortly after. I let go of a love that no longer existed. I had to face the facts that I couldn't change or mold someone into who I wanted them to be. They had to change for themselves. I experienced hurt and allowed people to mistreat me. I knew how I should have been treated. But, I did learn the grass is never greener on the other side.

Manipulation and deception come in all forms of shapes and sizes. I had ongoing destructive behavior by bringing the enemy closer to me. I allowed the enemy to sleep in my bed or enter into my world. After they slept well, they destroyed it and left it in shambles. They didn't know what loyalty meant. Loyalty isn't about how long you have known someone but how you treat them.

Everyone plays a role in your life. Some are there for one season and others for multiple seasons. I have watched seasons repeatedly change only to realize the ones who should've been here with me through the beautiful spring weather, summer nights, to watch the leaves falling off the trees, and the icy storms were not. I made peace with myself. I learned to humble myself while breathing in the fresh air. Forgiveness has replaced grudge in my vocabulary. I am finally accepting and embracing my beautiful skin, my beauty Wounds, and refers to myself as a warrior. The life lessons taught me to continue to fight and never give up on my dreams and success. My life may be turbulent, but there is a balance. I have shown no one can break me and that I am a warrior of all aspects. In Roman times the Greek goddess of wisdom and war was

The Journey of the Unbreakable Warrior

Athena. As I look in the mirror, I am her but instead of carrying her name, call me Phoenix Warrior.

The Journey of the Unbreakable Warrior

CPSIA information can be obtained
at www.ICGtesting.com
Printed in the USA
BVHW071931300921
617863BV00011B/407